SUDDEN INFANT DEATH (S.I.D.S.)
Probable Causes & Simple Prevention

SUDDEN INFANT DEATH (S.I.D.S.)

Probable Causes & Simple Prevention

James W. Tyler

Introduction by
Robert S. Mendelsohn, M.D.

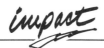

 Sterling Publishing Co., Inc. New York

Acknowledgments

To Les Winrow for his original art work.

To Dr. Steve Taylor for his ideas and for his lengthy, detailed criticism of my ammonia factor model.

To Jon Eisen, whose determination has enabled this book to be published.

Library of Congress Cataloging-in-Publication Data

Tyler, James W.
 Sudden Infant Death.

 (A Sterling impact book)
 Rev. ed. of: Cot death. 1983.
 Bibliography: p.
 1. Sudden death in infants. 2. Ammonia—Toxicology.
I. Tyler, James W. Cot death. II. Title.
III. Series. [DNLM: 1. Ammonia—poisoning—popular
works. 2. Sudden Infant Death—etiology—popular
works. WS 430 T982i]
RJ59.T95 1986   618.92   85-32325
ISBN 0-8069-6346-8 (pbk.)

Copyright © 1986 by James W. Tyler
Published by Sterling Publishing Co., Inc.
Two Park Avenue, New York, N.Y. 10016
Distributed in Australia by Capricorn Book Co. Pty. Ltd.
Unit 5C1 Lincoln St., Lane Cove, N.S.W. 2066
Distributed in the United Kingdom by Blandford Press
Link House, West Street, Poole, Dorset BH15 1LL, England
Distributed in Canada by Oak Tree Press Ltd.
% Canadian Manda Group, P.O. Box 920, Station U
Toronto, Ontario, Canada M8Z 5P9
Manufactured in the United States of America

1219

Table of Contents

Dedication

To my wonderful 92-year-old mother and her positive, supportive advice.
To my wife Miriam, for her patience and spirited, constructive ideas.
To my children, Timothy and Emily, who enabled me to make my crib observations.
And to all those families who have suffered the loss of a loved infant.

About This Book

For years, the spectre of a mysterious, sudden infant death has haunted parents all over the world. In the United States alone, more than 8,000 babies die every year, succumbing to "inexplicable" causes, alone at night in their crib. Their breathing "just stops."

This phenomenon, known as crib death or Sudden Infant Death Syndrome (S.I.D.S.), has stymied the medical profession for decades, despite millions of research dollars.

Long thought to be a killer virtually without any symptoms, S.I.D.S. strikes out at apparently healthy babies — babies who are loved, wanted, and apparently in competent hands.

One of these babies was Timothy Tyler, son of James W. Tyler, a New Zealand research biologist and lecturer. The baby was in good health when put to bed on a warm night in June, 1974, but some hours later, when Tyler went to check on him before retiring, he was overcome by the powerfully pungent odor of ammonia gas coming from the child's crib. Even more significant was the fact that the baby was strangely limp and colorless, and was having considerable trouble breathing.

Tyler immediately changed his diaper, and with some fresh air, little Timmy quickly revived.

This incident began 12 years of research for the elder Tyler whose findings, published here, are likely to start a major medical controversy.

Basically Tyler "discovered" something that every parent and pediatrician already knows: that there is ammonia in the baby's environment, and that this ammonia can and probably does cause a toxic reaction for whoever breathes it. For the young baby, with highly sensitive tissues, this reaction can be extreme.

Ammonia is a highly caustic gas, formed as a byproduct of the interaction between the urea in the urine and the *E. coli* bacteria in the stool. The diaper itself is the breeding ground for the production of this ammonia that is even toxic for an adult at only 50 parts per million.

Tyler writes, "It is remarkable that such a dangerous poison has never featured in any previous medical reference to crib death or infant death."

According to the Department of Environmental and Occupational Medicine at Mount Sinai School of Medicine in New York, Tyler is absolutely correct: There is ammonia in the crib, yet there has never been a study of potential toxins in the crib, including ammonia. Yet, in new Zealand at least, the head of the Cot Death Society, the group that funds research into S.I.D.S., went on record as saying that the ammonia theory was "old and discredited," although she later admitted to me that it was not. Nevertheless, the Tyler hypothesis, an obvious avenue to explore, has never been funded by the medical establishment, whereas projects focusing on prenatal brain dysfunctions and their potential relationship to S.I.D.S. have been.

Tyler's efforts — spanning 12 years — have been prodigious, and have attracted the attention of journals such as England's prestigious *New Scientist* (January 5, 1984). He has correlated every major and hundreds of minor S.I.D.S. studies with everything that is known about ammonia gas poisoning. He found that contrary to popular and medical myth, 84 percent of the S.I.D.S. babies have clear-cut, recognizable symptoms that an educated parent or pediatrician might well have heeded.

He found the "fingerprints" of ammonia gas poisoning in the autopsies of S.I.D.S. babies: glottal stenosis (constriction of the glottis, the opening between the vocal chords) pinpoint hemorrhaging of the esophagus, chemical pneumonitis (a chemically induced pneumonia) and even right ventricular enlargement of the heart.

This last finding is very important in the overall ammonia theory. Ammonia is not only a highly caustic substance, capable of inflaming the tissues of the respiratory system, it also combines with carbon dioxide in the bloodstream, and a baby needs *free* carbon dioxide to trigger the breathing reflex. If free CO_2 is not present in suitable quantities, the body is fooled into thinking it has enough oxygen, when in reality it is being starved of oxygen. There is ample indication that, in a large percentage of S.I.D.S. babies, there has been chronic hypoxia, or oxygen starvation.

Ever the deductive sleuth, Tyler has developed a sociology of S.I.D.S., in which he correlates S.I.D.S. cases with weather, socio-economic groupings, breast- versus bottle-feeding, and other factors that when taken together give a broad, overall picture of the syndrome.

8

According to Tyler, the medical community has appropriated a *problem* and in naming it, has created a new "disease" for which money must then be allocated in order to find a "cure." His point is that, over time many S.I.D.S. cases have been explained by better diagnoses or autopsies that show, say, heart dysfunctions. However, the solution to the mystery of the "unexplained" cases may lie in an area where establishment medicine has thus far refused to investigate.

—Jonathan Eisen
Editorial Director,
Sterling IMPACT Books

Introduction

S.I.D.S. will never be the same again! An unknown scholar from the end of the world has upstaged all the learned professors in all the prestigious medical centers by taking two sets of data and, with a master stroke of insight, showed their perfect fit. If intelligence is indeed the ability to recognize significant correlations, then J.W. Tyler qualifies as a genius.

On the one hand, we have a disease of unknown cause that has been studied to death. Doctors know when it occurs and in which population groups, and are aware of such incriminating factors as failure to breast-feed, low birth weight, diphtheria vaccine, and smoking during pregnancy.

On the other hand, doctors know the signs and symptoms of poisoning due to ammonia.

But, in their fruitless forays into physiology and in their empty search for viruses and bacteria, they have overlooked the possibility of a toxic etiology for the Sudden Infant Death (crib death) Syndrome. Unable to distinguish between simplicity and simplistic, medical researchers have ignored the insight of this uncredentialized yet wise thinker. But no matter, with this well-documented book, reflecting not only the brilliance, but also the sensitivity and compassion of its author, the genie is now out of the bottle.

Parents of S.I.D.S. victims, parents of infants sick from other diseases, and parents of healthy infants must read this book. They will then understand that the self-serving plea of S.I.D.S. researchers calling for more research money has been nullified by this revolutionary model for comprehending S.I.D.S.

Armed with this theoretical and practical tool, parents can begin to ask the necessary questions and take the necessary actions that will result in the first decreased incidence in history of this major killer of our infants.

Robert S. Mendelsohn, M.D.
Author of *Confessions of a Medical Heretic*

Preface

The book you are about to read espouses a very controversial theory concerning sudden, unexpected deaths in infancy, and prescribes an almost absurdly simple remedy for a problem that has gainfully employed thousands and worried millions more. According to the author, no one has taken it seriously. Why should you?

The lack of scientific recognition should be disturbing. It is the scientific community, however, more than Mr. Tyler, that disturbs me. Have we perhaps been overlooking the obvious all these years? Is this another case of pooh-poohing ideas that do not emanate from medical universities, but instead come from lay people or those not generally viewed as experts? In actuality, many advances in medical science have originated outside the scientific establishment, or sprung like Minerva from the head of some obscure thinker with no laboratory, no budget, and no friends in high places.

I frankly find Tyler's hypothesis logical and credible. As with any scientific theory, some aspects will undoubtedly be corroborated by and others contradicted by experimental evidence. But egg on one's face, as in "Why didn't I think of that," is a poor rationale for our evident reluctance to put the idea to the test. But isn't it "just too simple" to be true? The notion of washing one's hands in between autopsy and surgery was also once derided as nursemaid science, not really worth the attention of those with skill and training. At the risk of sounding like a retread politician, complexity and convolutedness need not always be virtues, nor simplicity inevitably a vice.

Purists may debate the merits of a hypothetical treatment or diagnostic technology, and this is arguably legitimate where the investment costs are high or the risks to health are palpable. But when neither is the case, arguments to avoid rocking the status quo are less convincing and, in our litigious times, the sniff of scientific disdain may be preferable to the taint of supposed indifference to the plight of victims.

In a nutshell, Tyler's proposition amounts to a sort of Toxic Shock Syndrome in diapers. He retraces the steps that led him to suspect environmental factors and point-by-point, shows how the properties and toxic effects of ammonia seem to match the surroundings and symptoms of crib death. Furthermore, he displays unusual sophistication for a layman in his treatment of ammonia as one member of a pluralistic matrix of causative and predisposing factors that are putatively operative in a surprisingly high number of infant sicknesses. He develops and proposes a conceptual pathology for both acute and chronic syndromes of ammonia toxicity, the former correlating with sudden infant deaths and the latter with not-so-sudden respiratory and gastrointestinal ills. Physicians will be interested in his review of the chronic physiologic effects of underventilation, as might be related to ammonia exposure. Transdermal absorption beneath *de facto* compression dressings in this age group may also be of clinical significance.

Supporters of breast-feeding will find an ally in this book. Tyler explains how ammonia concentrations and susceptibility to ammonia-related complications may be enhanced by formula feedings, and why the apparent immunity to S.I.D.S. during the first few weeks of life may in part be a function of the specialized neonatal metabolism of ammonia, a delicate balance that nutriment other than mother's milk may hazardously upset. I do not make my living from the practice of pediatrics, but I have been for some time sufficiently impressed by the available evidence that encourages colleagues to promote breast-feeding as a preferred alternative to bottled formulas.

Tyler also mounts a harsh critique of the official U.S. Public Health Service definition of S.I.D.S., which he believes stifles the pursuit of solutions. As he suggests, defining a condition by the absence of any demonstrable cause invariably seems to leave one holding an empty sack when it comes to researching and especially preventing the malady in question. It's similar to holding a race whose contestants are limited to those who do not enter.

I would not hesitate to show this book to expectant mothers. It just may prove lifesaving for families whose infants might have been lost while awaiting the results of formal investigation. Self-care augments medical care, and we physicians should continue to encourage it for our own betterment as well as for that of our patients.

Ultimately, a particularly susceptible subgroup of infants may be shown to exist, and means for early recognition may be developed. Tyler suggests that this may already be the case with low birth-weight babies, possibly caused by maternal smoking. Nevertheless, in the meantime, protective steps can and should be taken to guard all newborns from unrecognized and potentially toxic exposures in the home. Change the diaper frequently, even at night; breast-feed; don't smoke; and ventilate the room without chilling the baby.

Kenneth H. Kline, M.D.

Kenneth H. Kline, formerly of New York Hospital, is currently in a private practice emphasizing preventive medicine.

Chapter One

The Lethal Fallacy

The medical profession has defined a distinct category of infants who are Sudden Infant Death Syndrome (S.I.D.S.) or crib death victims. It has pursued this definition for more than 15 years.

However, this book will show that there can be no such separate syndrome, as the medical world presently defines it. Moreover, it will also show that the S.I.D.S. model of infant death causation is a lethal fallacy. It is a fallacy because it is a medical model that is philosophically untenable; it ignores contrary evidence; it is only sustained by statistical gerrymandering; and it has an implausible lack of correlation with the real causes of sudden infant death. The S.I.D.S. model focuses enormous research programs on discovering a *medical* solution to these infant deaths, and helps divert research from the reality of the environmental causal relationships to these deaths. Under this medical strategy, infants are dying needlessly, not from medical causes, but from *avoidable* environmental exposure trauma.

Until the publication of "Cot-Death: The Ammonia Factor" in 1983 (1), not one research article was ever published on a known, deadly respiratory poison that is potentially present at every infant's crib: ammonia gas.

There is no justification for the S.I.D.S. model created by the medical profession, but there are environmental factors that singly or in concert can cause infants to die. I will not dispute the fact that some infants die suddenly and from no apparent cause. On the other hand, I will dispute the theory that they die from some nameless, random disease syndrome that strikes without cause. Infants can and do die from exposure to an environmental stress trauma or a series of environmental stress traumas that can be symptomatologically nonspecific.

The medical research lobby has pressured the medical profession so skillfully that it actually believes the Sudden Infant Death Syndrome is a real *disease* which, with more time and money, will be revealed. Laymen do not have to believe in nonsense, but the longer they allow the medical profession to be deluded, the more reluctant it will be to believe it. And more infants will die needlessly.

Perhaps the problem can be put into perspective by looking at a related example. The New Zealand economy is quite dependent on its sheep industry. Thousands of farmers care for up to 70 million sheep. In a bad season, the total number of lambs marketed is considerably less than in a good season. This is because there are a lower number of births, as well as a higher death rate for the lambs that are born. Moreover, the farmer receives less money for the lambs that are sold because they are of poor quality. Many of the lambs that do not survive have died from nonspecific causes. They did not thrive. The sheep industry does not invest large amounts of research money trying to identify the various nonspecific causes of the higher lamb mortality in the bad seasons. It knows that it is the adverse combination of bad season conditions that is directly responsible for the losses. It recognizes that improving environmental conditions will lessen the death toll. Farmers also know that some sheep "races" or varieties withstand adverse conditions more successfully than others. They know that handing over large research funds to veterinarians will not lessen the toll of a bad season.

If lambs are analogous to infants and veterinarians to doctors, the doctors would get no special funding.

There are many environmental conditions that the sheep farmer cannot alter. However, the human race prides itself on its ability to improve and manipulate its environment. Is it surprising, then, that the statistics indicate that those nations with the most advanced and dedicated infant environmental care programs have the lowest overall infant death rate?

This book is the study of a known environmental hazard that is potentially present in every infant's crib. It is up every pediatrician's nose. And yet, it has never been the subject of any published study. It provides an environmental stress factor that is compatible with the total range of both pre- and postmortem infant death evidence, disproving the exclusivity of the medical profession's S.I.D.S. model of infant death causation.

My hope is that this book will help enable parents and governments alike to take positive, concerted steps in preventing the needless death of more of our children.

Chapter Two

An Infant's Ammonia Event

For 12 years, an incident has haunted me. Late one night, as I checked my sleeping infant son, my head was jerked back from his crib by the concentrated, pungent odor of ammonia gas. And yet my son was in a profound sleep. The ammonia that rocked my head had no such irritating effect on him. There was an unusual limpness about him and he didn't stir until I had changed his diaper. Like many parents, I had a dread and subconcious fear of crib death. The experience with my son and his ammonia-reeking diaper pointed to that highly poisonous chemical, ammonia, as a factor causing crib death. However, it is not an easy matter to change a sense of disquiet and foreboding into proven scientific evidence.

It has taken me a long time to come to terms with this problem. I have spent years working and watching my two children grow and flourish, while wondering how a case could be made against ammonia without any direct evidence except that brief encounter 12 years ago. So I began collecting information about ammonia and crib death — as much as I could find.

As the evidence against ammonia accumulated, the pressure increased to warn mothers about the dangers their infants faced from ammonia poisoning. I didn't feel any less pressure knowing that crib death, which was caused by this factor, could be so easily avoided.

The problems facing a layman trying to convert the medical profession to a new medical theory are so daunting, I have given up trying. The reactions have ranged from polite nods to patronizing put-downs to outright hostility. The standard reply (like the one I received from the poisons center when I raised the possibility of ammonia being a lethal agent in crib death) is that there is no hard evidence. When I tried to warn the *Australian Medical Journal* as long ago as 1975, I was told that the journal was not interested in reporting hypotheses. Because medical people are unwilling to venture into a discussion about a subject that isn't their specialty, the difficulty of trying to convince them is further compounded. In addition, as you get higher and higher up the specialty ladder, you eventually come face to face with the particular oracle in the particular specialty who turns out to have very definite views and with whom it is even more difficult to discuss something new.

When I tried to interest newspapers and other news media in what seemed to me to be a highly newsworthy and controversial item, I got a completely negative response. So my attempts have narrowed down to one final option: publishing the case myself against ammonia as a factor in infant death causation.

It's my intention in this book to convince people, especially mothers, that infant death causation is primarily an environmental problem and not primarily a medical problem. However, there are difficulties in trying to communicate with people when discussing medical research. The chief problem is that the precise terminology of medical research has to be translated into understandable, nonscientific language. All translations lose precision of detail in passing from one language to another. I hope my effort does not cause too many obscure meanings.

As for any doctor who reads this and wishes to dispute my case, my reply is that I have faced all kinds of objections to my arguments for the last 12 years. I have met very few doctors in that time who have been prepared to sit down and try to sort out the case against ammonia in a positive way. While I have been trying to get together the so-called hard evidence that is demanded, many infants have perhaps died needlessly. I do think I have reached a stage where the arguments are so convincing that I am prepared to present them to the people that matter: the mothers of infants at risk from ammonia poisoning. I challenge the doctor to produce a case that definitely proves that ammonia is not a factor in crib death.

Indeed the evidence that has become so clearly conclusive against ammonia as an agent in crib death has now pointed to a much wider target area: the group of infants who are reported as dying from acute, infectious respiratory diseases and, to a lesser extent, intestinal infectious diseases and other infectious and parasitic diseases.

The concepts of evidence and proof are at the heart of the legal, medical, and scientific professions. Repeatable evidence directly showing the actual crib death effect of ammonia on infants is impossible to secure. It is out of the question to deliberately expose infants to lethal chemicals. However, it is possible to reconstruct the effect of ammonia on the infant victim. Just as law officers carefully sift the site of a crime and obtain irrefutable evidence that can condemn a criminal after the event, it is also possible to go back to the scene of the crib death and point to the phantom presence of lethal ammonia that could have been present at the death scene. Just as police use a wide range of forensic tools including pathological examination in presenting their case, it is also possible to sift through the vast accumulation of pre- and post-death information, as well as environmental and sociological information, to determine that ammonia is indeed a phantom factor involved in crib deaths.

A common misconception is that the victims of crib death are perfectly normal babies who showed no symptoms of any looming tragedy. However, this is definitely not the case. The crib death victim suffers from a wide range of symptoms. So many in fact, that to attempt to link them and provide a single main cause of death has proved impossible up to the present.

A Sheffield, England, study from 1972–1976 showed that 97 children who had died from crib death had a total of 260 symptoms during the 3 weeks before death, whereas only seven were said to have been completely symptom-free for the whole period. (2)

Ammonia has a variety of effects on many life-sustaining systems. But since these effects vary with concentration exposure, it is a particularly difficult task to expose ammonia as the dangerous chemical it is. However, I will show that the varied effects of infant exposure to the poison gas ammonia are compatible with nearly all the known phenomena seen in crib death victims.

The bits of evidence of ammonia involvement are similar to the assorted pieces of a jigsaw puzzle. It is exceedingly difficult to fit together so many odd pieces in order to produce a clear picture. However, once I assembled the evidence, the final pattern highlighted ammonia as an obvious but overlooked environmental hazard whose lethality disproved a S.I.D.S. model of infant death causation. It supported instead a nonspecific environmental stress trauma model of infant death causation.

Chapter Three

The Pattern of Infant Death

According to the medical profession, a crib death victim can only be diagnosed as such if the infant, upon pathological examination, shows no inherently lethal pathology. To an ordinary person, such a definition is a contradiction in terms because a syndrome is a term usually applied to a group of symptoms occurring together and constituting a disease to which some particular name is given (3). The crib death syndrome definition specifies that if a disease is found, then the infant is not a crib death syndrome case. In a sense the medical research lobby has painted the medical profession into a corner by causing it to accept and officially recognize such a bizarre definition. Is it any wonder that many doctors have difficulty diagnosing a syndrome *whose definition is the absence of any syndrome or disease?* They have defined the conditions for a death group even though they don't know anything about the cause of the deaths.

What is the real pattern for sudden infant death?

Is Crib Death Genetically Determined?

Is the crib death factor inherited? Is it environmentally linked? Is it a minor genetic dysfunction that is triggered into a lethal effect by environmental factors? A number of studies have been carried out to detect whether crib death is directly inherited. To date no study has been able to show dominant, recessive, or sex-linked genetic characteristics in relationship to crib death. Peterson studied crib death's rate of incidence among first cousins. He showed that it was no higher than in the community as a whole. He also showed there was no difference in crib death rates between fraternal or identical twins (4). Beckwith showed that, although there was an increased risk for later offspring in families that had a crib death victim, the risk could not be ascribed to genetic inheritance (5).

A study by Spiers of twin deaths also noted that like-sexed and unlike-sexed pairs are equally affected. His results pointed to environmental factors being responsible for crib deaths (6).

In spite of a widespread search for a genetic link by these people and many others, none has been discovered. Moreover, a survey of a number of minor abnormalities, noted at birth in babies who subsequently became crib death victims, showed no evidence that sudden death babies had more oxygen deprivation, damage from anesthetic agents, or trauma before or during delivery than babies who did not die (4).

A final factor disproving a genetic cause of crib death is that these crib deaths occur within specific time spans. During the first 3 weeks of life, there is hardly any crib death. Between 2 and 3 months, there is a marked peak. After an infant reaches 5 months, crib death is extremely rare.

A further time constraint is indicated by the very name, crib death. It is confined to the hours of sleep. There is a specific and very brief time capsule in which crib death occurs and a more specific time constraint within the capsule itself. No genetic relationship has ever been demonstrated to be so specifically time controlled.

Not only did the studies trying to connect crib death to a genetic thread fail to do so, but by their very failure they pointed to environmental factors being the cause of crib death. The study on twins showed that the line of crib death to twinning could not be explained genetically. However, the rate of death among twins was many times higher than in the population as a whole. There had to be a shared environmental condition to account for the statistical difference. Although the answer was becoming obvious, the question still had to be asked.

Is Crib Death Environmentally Linked?

Although no dominant, recessive, or sex-linked genetic relationship can be established to explain crib death, there is still the possibility of a minor inherited trait being present that could be triggered by some environmental event. A number of minor dysfunctions have already been shown to have no genetic connection, but that study by no means exhausts the possibilities.

No matter what minor dysfunction is found to be capable of environmental triggering, the victims would be just part of a group who actually suffer crib death. Identification of such a group would point to the general area that the environmental factors work through in causing crib death. So it would be helpful if any such group could be identified.

The question still remains to be answered: Is there any evidence that links crib death to the environment?

The answer is yes—overwhelmingly yes. There is not just one environmental factor; there is a multitude of environmental links to crib death. The problem involves sifting through the enormous amount of environmental linkage to try to pinpoint specific factors acting through many environmental constraints. The next chapter summarizes main environmental factors found to be associated with crib death.

Chapter Four

The Environmental Factors Associated with Crib Death

Time of day—Crib deaths have always been associated with sleep. Typically the infant is put down to sleep and is later found dead. The infant is not observed and apparently dies silently and without struggle. By calculating the death time as midway between the moment the infant was last seen alive and the moment it was found dead, a study was able to show that 50 percent died from midnight to 8 a.m., 36 percent between 8 a.m. and 4 p.m., and 14 percent between 4 p.m. and midnight (7).

Time of year—There is a peak incidence of crib death during the winter months in both hemispheres. The crib death rate is independent of the seasonal variation in birth numbers. The main winter features found to relate most closely to crib death numbers are (1) a sharp temperature drop, (2) windspeed, (3) relative humidity, and (4) snowfall.

Time of life—Crib deaths occur within an extremely precise and narrow time frame. Most crib death victims are between 3 weeks to 1 year in age. There is a marked peak at 2 to 3 months. Crib death is extremely rare after 5 months of age. The most inexplicable feature of this time capsule is the apparent immunity infants have during the first 3 weeks of life.

Year of death—An intriguing feature noted recently is the statistical lessening of all infant death rates in a number of centers over a period of years. (7)

Place of death—Sweden would definitely be the place to live if you wished to avoid crib death. The rate there is reported as low as 0.6 for 1000 live births. (8) The rates vary from place to place. Ontario, Canada, had a reported 3 per 1000 live births (9) and in 1978–79, New Zealand had a rate of 2.2 for 1000 live births. (10)

Race of victims—A California study of 525 autopsied victims by Kraus (11) showed quite significant differences from that expected on the basis of proportional distribution of live births.

In New Zealand for the years 1970 to 1972 and 1978 to 1979, a similarly striking disparity was found between the crib death rate of European and Maori victims.

Table 1. Analysis of Crib Death Victims by Race,
California and New Zealand

Location of Death	Race of Victims	No. of Victims per 1000 Live Births
California	Oriental	0.51
(525 victims	White	1.31
in 1972)	Mexican	1.74
	Negro	2.92
	American Indian	5.93
New Zealand 1970–1972	European	1.5
	Maori	4.3
New Zealand 1978–1979	European	1.9
	Maori	4.0

An unusual feature of the New Zealand figures was the fact that there were 4.4/1000 live-birth Maori female victims against 0.7/1000 live-birth European (New Zealand) female victims. The death rate for Maori girl infants was more than six times the European rate (12). These figures differ considerably from several studies that have shown figures of 58–59 percent male, 41–42 percent female in five sets of figures (5), and a figure of 127 males/100 females for the United Kingdom (13).

Bladder state—This is both an environmental factor and a post-death symptom. The crib death victim is almost always found with an empty bladder. Infants who die from pneumonia, leukemia, or from other causes usually have a full bladder (14).

Birth weight of the infant—There is a consistent pattern of higher incidence of crib death associated with lower birth weights of infants. The death rate ranges from 0.8/1000 live births in those whose birth weight had been over 4500g (10 lbs.) and up to 6.55/1000 live births in those whose birth weights had been between 1500g (3.4 lbs.) and 2000g (4.5 lbs.) (15). Similar ratios have been found in New Zealand. The birth weight category of less than 2500g (6 lbs.) had a death rate of 6.8/1000 live births. That of the group with weight greater than 3500g (7.7 lbs.) was 2.0/1000 live births. (9)

24

Multiple births — If one twin died of crib death, the chance that the other will die from crib death is increased to between 5 and 8 percent regardless of whether the twin is identical or fraternal (4). This important study showed that a genetic link was most unlikely for crib death victims. However, the rate is still much higher than that in the general population. This is a definite pointer to an environmental link with crib death victims.

Family relationship — There is an increased risk of crib death occurring within a family that has already experienced a crib death. Like the twin study, the rate is much less than would be the case if the cause were of genetic origin. The figures point to an environmental factor increasing the risk for the remaining siblings (16). Froggatt's studies showed that the recurrence rate among siblings was between 11 and 22/1000 siblings at risk. This figure points very directly to an environmental factor being responsible for the increased vulnerability to the infant (14).

Infant feeding — There is a body of seemingly contradictory evidence surrounding the infant feeding factor. One study showed that infants who had soft pillows and were bottle-fed in the first 2 weeks of life showed a much higher rate (7.00/1000 live births) than those who had a hard pillow or none at all and were breast-fed only (0.60/1000) (13).

Froggatt, on the other hand, showed that the feeding histories of affected infants revealed almost identical feeding patterns for the victims and their matched controls. Froggatt also reported two victims who had been exclusively breast-fed (16).

A clear result showing the benefit of breast-feeding is given by a study done by Tonkin in Auckland. She reports that of 86 cases of crib deaths studied in Auckland, 83 were artificially fed and only three breast-fed at the time of death. A matched control showed 45 percent breast-fed at 2 weeks of age and 25 percent breast-fed at 3 months (12).

Illegitimacy — One survey found that 18 percent of the crib death cases were illegitimate, compared with 8 percent of a control group (13).

Crowded and unsanitary conditions — Statistics taken from a set of crib death victims showed that there are more people per room in crib death cases than in a control group studied at the same time. In addition to the overcrowding, more unsanitary conditions were found in the homes of the crib death victims than in the homes of the control group (13).

Socio-economic level — There is a higher incidence of crib death found among the lower socio-economic levels of society. It is highest among non-whites of lower socio-economic levels and it is higher among non-whites regardless of their socio-economic level (13).

25

Overheating — Overheating has been found to be associated with crib death events. The body temperature at death, the temperature of the environment at death, and excessive clothing are risk factors associated with overheating (17).

Age of the mother — Infants of young mothers seem more at risk from crib death than infants of mature women. In particular, women under 20 years of age who have had more than one child seem to have a greater vulnerability. The older the mother is, the less chance there seems to be for her infant to suffer crib death (16).

Smoking — Women who smoke during pregnancy directly affect the birth weight of their fetuses. There is a clear and proven connection between the degree of smoking done by the pregnant woman and the weight of the baby. The more smoking, the less the weight of the newborn. Low birth-weight infants (less than 2500g) (6 lbs.) are many times more prone to crib death than infants of higher birth weight (4000g) (8.6 lbs.) (18).

Prenatal education — Women who have received no prenatal care have significantly higher rates of crib death for their infants than mothers who have received regular prenatal attention.

Drugs and medical treatment — Methadone treatment for a pregnant woman in curing opium addiction has a very direct influence on raising the chance of crib death for her infant (19). Because cigarette smoking by a pregnant mother directly contributes to lowering the birth weight of her infant, the rate of crib death incidence automatically increases. It is perhaps not surprising that there are also increased rates of crib death found among the infants of women who smoke after birth.

There is a lack of information regarding a correlation between crib death incidence and the prescription drug treatment of pregnant women, mothers of newborn infants, and their infants. As drugs such as methadone and cigarette smoke have a high correlation with an increase in crib death, this is a worrisome information gap in the environmental knowledge associated with the causation of death through chemical means.

The effect of the economy on the infant mortality rate — The infant mortality rate in the United States is adversely affected by economic downturn, particularly by unemployment. In New Zealand the only periods when infant mortality failed to fall for each 5-year period this century were following the depression of the 1930s and in the 1970s. The post-neonatal mortality rate has remained stationary for the two 5-year periods of the 1970s (20).

26

Chapter Five

Summary and Analysis of the Environmental Factors

So far all the known factors associated with crib death that I have been able to find have been described. I will now list all these factors. From this list, an overview of crib death causes will emerge and a pattern will start to become evident.

1. Time of Day Link — At least 50 percent of crib deaths are from 12 p.m. to 8 a.m.

2. Time of Year Link — Winter is by far the most dangerous period.

3. Weather Links — Crib deaths are associated with:
(a) sharp temperature drop
(b) relative humidity increase
(c) snowfall
(d) low sunshine hours
(e) high wind speed
(f) little outdoor exposure

4. Geographical Link — Crib deaths occur more with:
(a) increasing latitude
(b) increasing population congestion
(c) regional outbreaks of respiratory disease

5. Day of the Week Link — No particular day is noted.

6. Sleep Link — Crib death is nearly always associated with babies who have been put down to sleep.

7. Duration of Sleep Link — Some deaths occur after only a very limited sleep period. Most occur late in sleep more than 5 hours after being put down.

8. Crib Link — Crib death victims are, as the name indicates, found dead in their cribs in most cases.

9. Racial Link — European races have much lower rates of crib death than non-European races for the same geographical areas. There has to be a specific genetic and environmentally linked factor responsible for this variation.

10. Sex Link — There is a marked excess in death rates for males.

11. Age Link — There is a peak of crib death at 3 months. It is most uncommon under 3 weeks of age. It is rare after 6 months of age.

12. Bladder State Link — Crib death infants are almost always found in wet diapers.

13. Birth-Weight Link — Low birth-weight infants have much higher death rates than heavy birth-weight infants.

14. Birth-Length Link — Short, low-weight infants have higher crib death rates than longer, heavier infants.

15. Position in Family Link — First-born babies are not as likely to suffer from crib death as later born brothers or sisters.

16. Family Link — Crib death rates are much higher for any infant if there has already been a crib death in the infant's family.

17. Twin Link — If one twin dies from crib death, regardless of whether it is an identical or fraternal twin, there is a higher than normal chance that the other will also die from it.

18. Infant Feeding Link — Totally breast-fed infants have less likelihood of crib death than infants who are not breast-fed.

19. Type of Birth Link — There are no figures on drug-assisted births, but there should be. The ordinary, normal birth complications do not increase the rate of crib death.

20. Sociological Link — The crib death rate is higher for the poor than for the well off, regardless of the race. The rate is higher among non-whites than whites, regardless of the income.

This extensive array of environmental factors can be tabulated as follows:

Table 2. Categories of Environmental Factors Associated with Crib Death

Category	Total Factors
Genetic	0
Environmental	38
Sex-related	2
Race-related	2
Maternal	15
Sociological	18
Time	12
Place	14
Baby's physical condition	16

This table highlights the major links to crib death. Moreover, it exposes a sobering reality: that there exists in our modern, so-called caring society a classical Darwinian struggle for survival for our infants that leads to a horrifying number of needless infant deaths.

In briefly viewing each category separately, certain points concerning this struggle become evident.

21. Bedding Link — Soft pillows are found to have a much higher association with crib deaths than hard, flat ones.

22. Housing Link — Infants living in overcrowded homes are more likely to suffer crib death than those who live in less crowded conditions.

23. Cleanliness Link — Infants living in unsanitary housing have higher death rates than those that live in sanitary conditions.

24. Post-birth Development Link — Infants who have poor overall physical development are more prone to crib death than normally developing infants.

25. Legitimacy Link — Illegitimate infants are much more prone to crib death than legitimate infants.

26. Age of Mother — Infants of mothers under 20 years of age are most vulnerable.

27. Smoking Link — Crib deaths are closely related to how much the mother smokes during and after pregnancy. The more she smokes, the more her chances increase for a crib death.

28. Prenatal Education Link — Women who have received no prenatal care have higher incidences of crib death in their infants than those who have received regular prenatal care.

29. Drug Link — There is an information gap on the effect of drugs, before, during, and after birth for mother and infant. There is a direct relationship between methadone-treated pregnant women and their infants' crib death liability. Drugs that would influence sleep state or fluid control (e.g. alcohol and antihistamines) seem to have a marked effect on crib death rates.

30. Economy Link — Severe downturns in the economy are reflected in higher crib death rates in the years following the downturns.

31. Temperature Link — There are environmental temperature, body temperature, and excessive clothing links.

Sex and Race Categories

This grouping is the odd one out in the category relationships. But it is highly significant because of the number of crib deaths in each category. The non-European (non-Caucasian) sections of each community have a much higher total crib death number per 1000 live births than Europeans (Caucasians) living in the same geographical locations.

It would seem that, apart from the normal spread of factors contributing to crib death among non-European infants, there is some other factor present that makes non-European infants much more vulnerable to crib death than European infants. I certainly do not agree with one doctor who casually brushed aside the importance of such a discrepancy with a callous, most unprofessional remark, indicating that Maori mothers don't really want their infants or care for them. In a way this was a turning point for me because I was being dismissed for my ammonia theory in the same offhanded manner. Just as there was no scientific support for such an unwarranted attack on the Maori, I also have realized that there was no scientific backing for a number of arguments that have been raised against my theory. Furthermore, does this dismissal of the Maori also extend to blacks and North American Indians for they have similar figures? The figures call for much greater investigation. Of course, such investigation would have been initiated and carried out until a solution were found had the figures been the other way around. The Maori love of family and race and indeed all races is there. It is real. My family and I live with it daily. There have to be other factors responsible for such a high and specific vulnerability of their infants to crib death than lack of love and care for their infants.

The Mother

As could be expected, the mother factor in crib deaths is emphasized by the number of factors associating her with it. Again the picture, drawn by the factors relating to her, is one of a woman under stress in a modern society. Is it any wonder that the woman — who is the most under stress from her youth and who has the burden of having an illegitimate infant, the burden of having several children close together, the burden of close living and unsanitary conditions, and the burden of economic stress — should face the highest risk for her infants? Added to this list is the problem of inadequate prenatal care. Is she struggling so desperately economically, that she can't find time to visit a prenatal clinic — or is the attitude she finds at such a clinic so repulsive to her that she refuses to attend? As health care for pregnant women in New Zealand is free, her unacceptance of it is worthy of investigation. As for health care: The cost of constant health care for her newborn infant is far too high. To go to the doctor about problems such as sniffles, change in cry, irritability, vomiting, diarrhea, sleeplessness, coughing, rash, and fever would be far too expensive. However, these symptoms are the signature of crib death. Is it all that surprising that the country with most support for its mothers is also the country with the lowest crib death rate? A caring system that would be acceptable to the mother would be able to detect problems arising for the baby and mother.

Sociological Factors

The main implications relating to the sociological factors influencing crib death have been dealt with in the previous category. Little more needs to be written, except for emphasizing that there is an undeniable relationship between the socio-economic status of a family and its rate of crib death.

Time and Place

Both time and place factors are highly important in crib death figures. There is a very distinct and clear relationship between the environmental factor(s) associated with causing S.I.D.S. and the timing and place of death.

Physical Condition of the Baby

The undersized baby with oxygenation problems due to its mother's heavy smoking and who is in a family situation of great stress is most vulnerable to crib death. This pattern of vulnerability is seen in the statistics which show that the same set of conditions that claim one infant in a family make it much more likely that another infant from the same family will also be claimed.

There seems to be optimum environments where the crib death rate falls to as low as 0.5/1000 live births. However, given poor environmental circumstances, the crib death rate reaches more than 10 times the base level. So there is an enormous potential for lowering the rate of crib death among infants at risk.

The lack of activity that would bring about a decrease in the environmental factors associated with crib death is hard to justify. It becomes even harder to justify when compared with the considerable research being done to determine physiological factors causing crib death. If a comparable series of studies on road accidents identified specific places where fatal accidents occurred due to a variety of environmental factors, it would be an obvious misdirection of resources if the authorities spent large sums of money sifting through vehicles searching for minor defects and took no action on the obvious environmental causes of the accidents.

Chapter Six
The Medical Question: Crib Death
Syndrome Symptoms

Not only is the standard definition of crib death philosophically untenable, it requires the absence of any verifiable cause of death after pathological examination. It is a definition that allows for no solution.

Moreover, there is a positive disincentive to find any specific cause. Because the definition gives no direction, any research must by definition be random. Because the absence of cause provides the tag of a positive, accepted death report, there is then the added disincentive for the pathologist or the coroner to pursue any investigation thoroughly. Because there is overwhelming evidence associated with sudden infant deaths, such evidence must be ignored because the definition of the syndrome demands that there is no solution.

The New Zealand public was given an instance of this behavior shortly after a radio program announced details of a *New Scientist* article on the ammonia factor theory (21). The official spokesperson for the Health Department advised mothers over national radio news to ignore the possibility of ammonia being a factor in causing crib death *even if a parent were to find its infant dead and smelling of ammonia.* This advice makes one wonder what other known, deadly relationships might be deliberately ignored.

Is it any wonder that, in the light of such an extraordinary definition, there is so much divergence of opinion between doctors on crib death events that they have diagnosed?

An example of how this classification is clouding the crib death numbers can be found in the work of the committees that reviewed the reported cause of death of the 310 post-neonatal deaths in New Zealand in 1978 through 1979. Initially 112 crib death cases had been reported out of the 310 post-neonatal deaths using the rigid international coding. The review committee considered that 154 deaths were classifiable to S.I.D.S. This is an increase of 37 percent over the initial number reported.

A further indication of the confusion over definition would seem to be behind the very marked difference in the proportions of total deaths classified as S.I.D.S. by the various committees.

Table 3. Total Post-Neonatal Death Numbers and the Percentage of Crib Death Cases by Health District

Health District	Total Deaths	Percent Crib Deaths	
Christchurch	44	70	
Dunedin	19	63	
Auckland	20	55	
Wellington	25	44	
South Auckland	22	41	
Hamilton	31	36	(9)

In an offhanded comment, a New Zealand demographic data report perhaps revealed the truth when it stated, "The increase in reported cases from sixty-seven to one hundred and seventy-nine over the period was probably an indication of the growing use of the term cot-death [crib death]" (22).

Rather than finding an increased number of crib death cases, a British government commission examination of reported deaths found exactly the opposite. It stated that the number of crib deaths reported was exaggerated. In a study of 988 deaths of babies between one week and two years of age in eight different British cities, it found that only 19 percent of the deaths were genuinely unexpected (23).

If such reviews come up with such grossly disparate results, then research that has been based on such subjective death reporting must be highly suspect.

Just as the study of the environmental factors associated with crib death produced a large number of seemingly unconnected factors, so also does a study of the symptoms of crib death. There is a large range of sublethal, nonspecific symptoms found in crib death victims. I will now examine these symptoms in two main groupings: pre-crib death symptoms and postmortem symptoms.

34

Pre-Death Symptoms

The extent of the number of symptoms that S.I.D.S. victims exhibit is highlighted by the Sheffield study. According to this study, the 97 crib death children had a total of 260 symptoms, and only seven children were completely symptom-free during the 3 weeks before death. Infants who have one or two of the following — sniffles (obstruction of the nose as indicated by noisy breathing whether or not accompanied by discharge), cough, irritability, vomiting, diarrhea, sleeplessness, rash, change of cry, and fever — are much more prone to crib death than infants without these symptoms. Indeed, the probability of death increases markedly if two or more symptoms are present, and the probability increases by a factor of three when sniffles accompany any other symptoms (2). During the last 3 weeks of life, 80 of the 97 infants who died had symptoms at the time of death and only seven were reported to have had none during the 3 week period. As much as 84 percent of the victims had more than one symptom. A control group had only 24 percent with one symptom and only 10 percent with more than one symptom (2).

Another recent work on 33 near-miss infants showed that 18 of the cases demonstrated signs suggesting that obstruction of air into the lungs was occurring in the upper-breathing spaces. All of those infants who showed the signs could only breathe through their nose (24). It seems that nearly half of all infants at 6 weeks can only breathe through their noses (25).

An earlier study using controls shows that 68 percent of S.I.D.S. victims had symptoms of respiratory infection, as compared with 32 percent of the controls. Just 2 percent had symptoms of gastric infection only, as against 0 percent in the controls. Only 20 percent of the crib death victims had no symptoms, compared with 61 percent of the controls (26).

Another observation made of a near-miss crib death victim was the altered pattern of dopa, dopamine, serotonin, and other amines in the infant's urine after the event (27).

Studies also show that the majority of sudden death babies had less intense reactions to various environmental stimuli than their surviving siblings had at the same age (4).

The apnea hypothesis was developed by Steinschneider, who reported prolonged periods of apnea during the sleep of several infants who later became victims of crib death. This finding focused attention on the respiratory system and its regulation (28). Apnea is described as arrested breathing. Children who are apparently normal occasionally stop breathing for as long as 40 seconds, then recover spontaneously, and seem none the worse for the spell.

Near-miss infants have been noted with abnormally low heart beat, as well as being apneic and cyanotic (29).

Apnea may be brought about by the control of the respiratory center through a stimulus or failure, or it may be mechanically induced through an obstruction. Although it is a possible cause of crib death, four out of five sudden deaths arose in children with no history of previous apneic attacks (30).

A variety of neurological abnormalities have been observed more frequently among future victims of crib death than in a set of matched controls. They include jitteriness or tremulousness, an abnormal Moro reflex, generalized muscular hypotonia, abnormal reflexes, and spontaneous hypo- or hyperthermia. These differences are statistically significant (31).

Postmortem Symptoms

The first thing to be noted about crib death babies is that, upon examination, their bodies appear to be well developed and well nourished (29).

The search for the basic cause of crib death can be narrowed by eliminating several very important factors.

Sudden death in adults is most often cardiac in origin and it specifically involves alteration in the rhythm of the heart beat (terminal arrhythmia). It is understandable that a similar cause would be sought for crib death. However, much investigation has produced evidence that shows that this is not the case. Of course, in the end, the heart has to stop beating, but there is evidence to show that the heart is beating right to the very end and it only stops because the S.I.D.S. baby has ceased functioning. A series of postmortem studies of crib death victims shows that the oxygen tension in the left heart has been found to be consistently low, suggesting that the heart beat continued after respiration ceased (32).

A further series of autopsy studies of crib death victims shows that a very high percentage of blood was completely unclotted in S.I.D.S. victims, and this was thought to point to continued movement of blood through tissues under profoundly hypoxic (low oxygen) conditions (33).

So the evidence, which shows that heart malfunction is not a primary cause of death in crib death victims, at the same time focuses on lack of oxygen and respiratory problems as factors in crib death (30).

36

Infection

Nearly 50 years ago, the first proven cause of sudden death in infants was published. Farber diagnosed massive streptococcal infection in infants who had died of sudden death (34). Later research shows that this was a relatively rare event and not a major cause of crib death. It is ironic to note that, under the present classification of crib death, those deaths examined by Farber would not even be reported as crib deaths.

Viral infections could play some role in S.I.D.S. Studies have shown a variety of viral readings in crib death cases ranging from 0 to 100 percent in the cases examined. The common history of respiratory infections and postmortem findings of inflammation in the upper respiratory tract indicated a viral relationship with crib death (29).

Underventilation

Following the development of the apnea theory by Steinschneider, Naeye recognized that severe underventilation would leave anatomical markers in infants who suffered from it. He did a series of postmortem studies, which show that most crib death victims suffered from underventilation and that there was a very wide spread of anatomical markers in these victims pointing to this underventilation (31).

In a comparison of 124 victims and 375 matched controls, Naeye and Dage found that the mean body weight, body length, and head circumference development of the victims had shown less growth than the controls. The growth delay involved bones, the brain, and other organs (35).

A more detailed tissue study by Naeye found that about 60 percent of the victims had abnormal pulmonary artery muscle and cardiac right ventricles. This was further supporting evidence of chronic underventilation.

Naeye further reasoned that the underventilation that produces such clear markers in the victims would also cause a low level of oxygen in the arterial blood that circulates through the rest of the body (hypoxemia) and that this should be able to be traced by its effect on body tissues.

He found that nearly half of the crib death victims had abnormal retention of brown fat. This is also found in infants who are chronically hypoxemic after birth. So this seems to indicate that the crib death victims also had long periods of low-level oxygen saturation in their blood.

Another tissue abnormality found in most crib death infants was an increased amount of the specialized adrenal gland tissue that makes adrenalin. The amount of brown fat in the body is controlled by the level of adrenalin in the blood.

Most of the crib death infants Naeye examined were producing red blood cells by the liver and they also showed an increase in the production of red blood cells in the bone marrow (32). Normally the liver doesn't make red blood cells after the first week of life. Both of these factors are signs of chronic low oxygen level in the blood. The hormone cortisone is found in high levels in crib death victims. The level normally rises in response to hypoxemia and other forms of stress.

Naeye's group also found that more than half of the crib death victims they studied had underdeveloped carotids. They play an important role in the reflex arousal out of rapid eye-movement (REM) sleep and in the switching on of the brain-stem mechanisms that restart breathing. Carotids are chemoreceptors, which being sensitive to chemical changes in the blood, protect it from lack of oxygen.

Naeye searched for symptoms of low-oxygen uptake in the brain. He found that about half of the crib death infants had abnormal amounts of the brain-stem tissue responsible for respiratory control. He claimed that this growth was not a cause of the low-oxygen level but a result of it (4).

Emery and Gadson have found that about half of the crib death infants they have studied have scavenger cells laden with fat in the spinal fluid (36). The fat appears to be derived from broken-down brain tissue. Chronic low-oxygen levels could be the cause of the broken-down tissue (33).

Supporting evidence possibly links this work on neutral fat in the brains of crib death infants to pre-death behavior which shows that many of the victims had less intense reactions to their environment than normal babies. It could also be possibly linked to subtle brain damage found in a number of crib death victims. There appears to be differences in the fatty insulation around two areas of the brain stem in a number of crib death victims. These areas are those that control respiration and other body functions (4).

A very disturbing feature of crib death for many parents is the presence of bloody, frothy fluid coming from the nostrils and mouth of their dead infant. Sometimes the fluid is only slightly blood tinged and sometimes it is simply a grey-white, frothy fluid. Not all children who die from crib death have this feature (37).

The other external features of crib death infants are cyanosis of the lips and nail beds. (Cyanosis is a bluish tinge shown by hypoxic tissue observed most frequently under the nails, lips, and skin. It is always due to lack of oxygen (38).

There is almost always an empty urinary bladder found in crib death victims (20). This has been noted earlier.

Petechiae or spot hemorrhages are usual in crib death victims. They are found throughout the upper breathing organs and right through the lung membrane and under the membrane of the heart. They are often so severe on the thymus and its membrane sac that they give a measly appearance to it. The larynx and vocal cords are also often found to have lesions and to be inflamed. Surface tissue is locally destroyed. The tiny abcesses are quite deep in the laryngeal tissue. The trachea usually has similar damage to the larynx and its surface cells are often shed (37).

Congestion and moderate edema are often noted in the lungs, usually filling the pleural cavities completely.

Occasionally edema of the vocal cords is noted. Edema is an abnormal infiltration of tissue with fluid (37).

The stomach of crib death infants usually contains undigested curd. Some thrown-up stomach curd is sometimes sucked into the larynx and trachea (7).

Chapter Seven

Summary and Analysis of the Pre- and Post-Mortem Symptoms

By its very definition, crib death victims can show no specific symptom that would cause death. For example, evidence of any overwhelming viral or bacterial infection would cause the death to be reported as such rather than as crib death. However, crib death victims still show a large number of common symptoms. As with the environmental factors, these symptoms can be put into categories.

Separate Element Symptoms
1. The infant is generally well developed and well nourished. However, studies show that the mean body weight, length of body, and head circumference are in general less than average. The victims do not tend to develop as well as normal infants.
2. The bladder of crib death victims is usually empty.
3. The victim is found to have had a fever or to have been irritable.
4. There are more male than female victims.

Intestinal Symptoms
1. Victims typically have curd in their stomachs.
2. They are often found to have suffered from diarrhea, rash, or vomiting in the 3-week period before death.

Neurological Symptoms
1. Victims tend to have shown less intense reactions to their environment than normal.
2. Victims are found to have suffered from jitteriness, an abnormal Moro reflex, muscular hypotonia, abnormal reflexes, and spontaneous hypo- or hyperthermia.

Breathing and Respiratory Symptoms of the Mouth, Nose, and Throat

1. Frothy, bloody fluid is often found coming from the mouth and nostrils of the victims.
2. Many victims have small hemorrhages throughout the upper respiratory organs.
3. There are often small, but deep, abscesses found in the laryngeal and pharyngeal tissue.
4. The victim is often found to have suffered from sniffles, coughing, and change of cry during the period preceding death.
5. There is evidence of pharyngeal airway obstruction in a number of infants.
6. Apnea episodes are of common occurrence.
7. The victim is often found with cyanosis of the lips.
8. Congestion and edema of the lungs is frequently found in crib death victims.

Table 4. Categories of Symptoms Associated with Crib Death

Category of Symptom	Total Symptoms
Single element symptom	4
Intestinal	2
Neurological	2
Mouth, nose, throat, and respiratory organs — breathing	8
Low oxygenation	10

Symptoms of Low-Oxygen Level in the Body

1. There is evidence of the heart beating after respiration ceased due to a very low oxygen blood level.
2. Unclotted blood is found in the heart after death. It is due to an extremely low oxygen level in the blood.
3. An abnormal amount of pulmonary arterial muscle, due to low-oxygen level, is found.
4. The cardiac right ventricles are overdeveloped due to chronic low-oxygen level.
5. There is brown fat retention due to chronically low oxygen levels.
6. There is larger than normal adrenal tissue that is used to control brown fat levels. This is a sign of low-oxygen level.

7. The cortisone level is abnormally high because of low-oxygen level and other forms of stress.

8. There is an abnormal amount of brain-stem tissue. The brain-stem tissue is responsible for respiratory control. The development is ascribed to a reaction to low-oxygen levels.

9. Scavenger cells are found laden with fat in the spinal fluid. A chronically low level of oxygen is given as the cause of this happening.

10. There are underdeveloped carotid bodies. These are usually underdeveloped in those cases that are found to be underventilating.

Chapter Eight

An Obvious Conclusion

A close examination of the literature on the major post-neonatal infant death groups reveals that in each group the apparent presentation of symptoms is even under dispute. An extensive United Kingdom survey (23) found that the suddenness factor in sudden infant death was present in *less than one fifth* of the cases where it was supposed to be. Also, those infants, reported as dying from respiratory disease or from gastrointestinal disease, upon pathological examination, typically had insufficient pathogens to have caused the deaths the infants were reported as having died from.

The medical research lobby would like the world to believe that their S.I.D.S. model of infant death causation allows it room to maneuver. This is not the case. This model is specifically concerned with an agent of death that is untraceable — that strikes suddenly, randomly, and unexpectedly. It is a syndrome that allows no near misses because it is only applicable to dead infants. Its defining parameters encompass a concept of lethality that is outside all the known death causation realities of medical history. It has neither predictive, diagnostic, protective, or preventive elements. *It is, indeed, the antithesis of the scientific model.*

Any sustainable model of infant death causation should provide predictive, diagnostic, protective, and preventative elements. It has already been found that countries that provide an intensive, environmental protective shield for their infants also dramatically lessen the numbers of infant deaths. Moreover, this is across the total spectrum of post-neonatal infant mortality, not merely the S.I.D.S. cases. This mortality decrease corresponds with the pattern of infant death revealed by the profile of environmental factors and by the pre- and postmortem symptoms. Although these countries have not precisely pinpointed the specific nature of the cause of those deaths, nevertheless, by putting a protective shield into place in the form of environmental care, they have effectively prevented the deaths of many infants through exposure to nonspecific environmental stress trauma.

Chapter Nine

The Toxic Profile and
Properties of Ammonia

Ammonia is potentially present at every infant crib because the urea that's excreted in urine is inherently unstable and is easily converted into ammonia through bacterial action.

Ammonia is a tissue-destroying, poisonous gas. It is colorless and basic.

It is highly soluble in water, forming ammonium hydroxide — a corrosive, alkaline substance. The pH of a one percent solution in water is 11.7.

Ammonium hydroxide differs from other alkalis in its volatility. The vapor (NH_3), even in low concentrations, is extremely irritating to the respiratory passages and the skin.

It has a low vapor density (0.59) relative to air (= 1). Ammonia is readily produced from urea. It has a pungent odor and is severely irritating to the membranes of the nose, throat, and lungs. Ammonia readily reacts with acid anhydrides. For instance, ammonia combines with carbon dioxide in the presence of water.

Part of the ammonia reaching the alveoli is neutralized by the carbon dioxide and part may be absorbed unchanged into the circulation. Ammonia acts principally on the upper respiratory tract with an alkaline, caustic action.

Ammonia causes saliva to be released and secreted.

Ammonia has a more corrosive local action on the tissues than do most acids.

Ammonia combines with tissues to form chemicals called albuminates and with natural fats to form soaps. Tissues are gelatinized to form soluble compounds and by so doing may produce deep and painful destruction of tissue. Soaps can act as free alkalis themselves to irritate tissue.

When first met, atmospheres slightly poisoned with ammonia are quite irritant, but the effect soon becomes less noticeable. Workmen frequently are found working without concern in an atmosphere that causes coughing and painful throat and nasal irritation in a person not used to the exposure.

The most dangerous consequence of exposure to ammonia gas is pulmonary edema. This occurs because of damage to the microvascular membrane. Acute damage causes increased microvascular permeability. Under this circumstance, edema may form with great rapidity (39).

Chemical pneumonitis is often produced in the lungs of people who have been exposed to ammonia. Chemical pneumonitis and pneumonia have a similar effect on people. However, with pneumonitis, there is no infection, and pneumonitis can result in death.

Ammonia may cause sensitization. A swallowed ammonia solution inflames the stomach, especially the mucous membrane lining the stomach.

Ammonia produces a narrowing of the tubes of the internal organs. It produces gastric, duodenal, and jejunal stenosis. (Stenosis means narrowing.) Increased absorption by the body of the ammonium ion can produce flaccid facial muscles, tremor, impairment of motor performance, and coma. A set of most interesting experiments with mice using intravenous ammonium ions produced a series of muscular contractions and relaxations, with rapid deep breathing and gasping. This was usually followed by profound coma. Death was preceded by convulsions. Survivors made a complete and rapid recovery.

Ammonia can produce sensations of suffocation caused by producing spasms of the glottis as well as by laryngeal edema. Vomiting may follow the laryngeal or glottal spasms.

Ammonia can produce long-term chronic irritation of the nose and upper respiratory tract. Ammonia inhalation causes chronic bronchial catarrh (inflammation of the bronchial mucous membrane over a long period, with a constant flow of mucus). It causes laryngitis and bronchitis. It also produces respiratory reflexes such as coughing and even respiratory arrest.

Ammonia causes death in a variety of ways. By far the most common cause of death from ammonia poisoning is pulmonary edema. It can also cause respiratory spasm with rapid asphyxia and coma. Respiratory arrest through reflex action and death follow. Ammonia also can affect the heart and cause cardiac arrest.

It is indeed a most hazardous chemical. Any amount of ammonia exposure can be dangerous (40, 41, 42).

Ammonia has been used medically as a heart stimulant (3).

The most worrisome aspect of the previous description of ammonia and its toxic pathways is that it is a description of the known and observed effects on adults. How much more dangerous must this poison be for the infant with its tender respiratory system?

Chapter Ten

The Case Against Ammonia

The case against ammonia is ready. All the evidence associated with the environment and the pre- and postmortem conditions of the infant victims has been assembled and tabulated. Also a profile of the known poisonous effects on humans from the chief suspect, ammonia, has been made. All that remains is to show, beyond all reasonable doubt, that the environmental categories and the pre- and postmortem symptoms are compatible with ammonia poisoning. The *modus operandi* pattern of criminal activity is a well-known tool used by police in obtaining convictions. I shall show that the *modus operandi* of ammonia is compatible with the whole bizarre range of environmental factors and with the pre- and postmortem symptoms found with crib death victims. The most frequent accusation levelled at my work is that I have no hard evidence. I deny this. I have assembled two complete sets of hard evidence, which has been published by reputable and distinguished scientists in a wide variety of medical journals and scientific texts. Basically all the ammonia factor theory does is relate together these sets of hard evidence. The fact that they relate together over such an enormous range of symptoms reinforces the relationship between both sets of information.

The Sleep Requirement for Ammonia Poisoning

Ammonia is potentially available, every day, with every infant, through the breakdown of the urea in its urine to ammonia. Urea is a naturally unstable compound, and slight heat moisture and bacteria cause it to break down to ammonia quite rapidly. To cause a buildup of ammonia for the infant, a prone position, at rest, for a period of time, is required. Because of ammonia's odor, the alert, awake baby would not tolerate irritating concentrations. So sleep is also a requirement for ammonia poisoning. It is a matter of statistics that babies are asleep, prone, and left unattended for the longest period between midnight and 8 a.m. It is a statistical fact that most crib deaths occur during that period.

The quantity of ammonia produced from the urine is dependent on the volume of urine, on its urea concentration, and on the presence of bacteria that will cause the ammonia to be released.

The Production of Ammonia

The output of urine by the newborn baby is dilute because the kidneys are immature at birth. The newborn infant passes 30 to 60 mL per day, for up to about 4 days. By the tenth day, the infant will pass about 10 times per day with a total output of from 100 to 300 mL of pale yellow urine. The frequency and amount of urine changes as food is increased. At 2 months, the amount voided is from 350 to 450 mL per day (43, 44). So there is a natural limitation to the urea available for degradation for at least the first week after birth. Ammonia would probably not be able to be produced in quantity for another reason in those early days.

It takes about a week for the newborn infant to adjust to food passing through. The first stool is a greenish-black one made up of debris swallowed in utero combined with shed cells, mucus, and other intestinal secretions. From about the fourth to the seventh day, there is a transition from this to greenish slimy stools. This is the changeover to milk stools. By the end of the first week, the infant will normally pass two or three milk stools per day (45).

At this point we come across the danger of artificial feeding. Sometimes it might come earlier, if the baby has supplementary feeding at night to ensure that the mother has a good night's sleep. But for a large percentage of babies, artificial feeding is a reality after 2 or 3 weeks. Sooner or later, for most babies, artificial feeding becomes a problem. There are all sorts of complications introduced to the digestive tract and to the metabolic systems of the infant by diet change. The digestive tract of the newborn infant is designed to deal with human milk. Nearly always it is quite able to thrive and grow on this diet without any other form of feeding for up to 6 months. The human digestive tract at the newborn stage of life is not developed to cope with artificial foods, cow milk, or infant formula milk. Any change in the amino acid balance in the composition of the infant diet could cause changes in the amount of urine excreted and an alteration of the urine composition — particularly in the concentration of urea excreted. Moreover, apart from altering the urea concentration, there are a number of other problems caused by artificial feeding.

Nearly all infant gastroenteritis victims are victims of artificial feeding. Infants who are breast-fed do not suffer gastroenteritis deaths to anywhere near the same degree as those who are artificially fed.

The antibodies in human milk alter the risk of infection in the baby. This antibody activity is not confined to the initial colostrum feeding of the infant, but extends to the milk. For as long as the baby is fed directly by breast, this risk of infection is reduced by these antibodies. They act locally in the gut and help with the breakdown of *E. coli* bacteria so that there is a lower risk of gastroenteritis. There is much less bacteria in the stools as a result. Essential fatty acids cannot be made by humans. They get them from their diet. The mother has some linoleic acid from her diet in her milk. With breast-fed babies, therefore, the concentration in the blood is about three times higher than that in bottle-fed babies. Linoleic acid is used in making cortisone (44).

Recently attention has been drawn to the possibility that various plant toxins contained in the feed of the cow are passed through its milk to the human consumer (45). It is well-known that many non-Europeans have great difficulty in digesting cows' milk. Perhaps it is a cow-milk reaction that accounts for the greater rate of crib death in non-Caucasians. Due to the gastrointestinal and growth problems caused by artificial feeding in infants of Papua, New Guinea, legislation was introduced to limit sales of bottles and nipples to those who were given a doctor's prescription.

A number of studies show that the crib death rate is closely related to artficial feeding rates. Of 86 cases of crib death occurring in Auckland in 1971 through 1973, 83 were artificially fed and only three breast-fed at time of death. This compared with a breast-feeding rate among controls of 45 percent at two weeks of age and 25 percent at three months of age (12).

Through artificial feeding, an imbalance is introduced to the gut and to the body metabolism. Urea excretion rates are altered with this unnatural loading. And because the natural antibodies present in breast milk are not there to protect the infant, infection flourishes. The feces become loaded with bacteria. The bacteria react with the altered urea concentration producing abnormal quantities of ammonia.

The Inhalation of Ammonia

Factors that influence the amount of ammonia inhaled by the infant are the air temperature, the relative humidity, the air movement, the crib design, the distance the ammonia has to travel, and the sleep pattern of the baby.

There is a specific set of climatic conditions that lead to increased vulnerability of the infant to crib death. That same set of conditions also leads to maximum ammonia exposure for the infant.

Convection currents play a large part in ammonia exposure. The colder it is, the more distinct the convection current will be. A convection current is formed when hot air rises and cold air falls. In an enclosed crib such a convection current would be easily set up under conditions of great temperature difference between the infant and the air. Such a convection current would require still air in an enclosed room. These conditions are most applicable in the winter months. The time and weather conditions are also those experienced in the formation of mists and fogs. The relative humidity, time, and weather conditions most noted for crib death relate to this set of mist and fog formation conditions. Being a low-density gas relative to air, ammonia would tend to escape more rapidly under other sets of conditions. Hence, this is a likely cause for the relationship of crib death to latitude and to seasons.

The inhalation of ammonia is increased by increased exposure to it. Such an exposure pattern relates to crib time. The infant — particularly in winter — is put down and left for long periods. An empty bladder with wet diapers is a feature of nearly all crib deaths. Longer periods of exposure to ammonia fumes are caused because the bacteria has a longer time to act on urea to produce ammonia and the baby is asleep and unattended for a longer time.

Dosage and Toxicity

Ammonia is an extremely toxic substance. But unlike a poison such as cyanide where a very small dose has invariably fatal results, the same cannot be said of ammonia. Its effects are quite variable. In describing these effects, the first thing to be done is to clarify the terms of dosage.

- Acute: refers to a sudden, or severe and short-lived, dose.
- Subacute: refers to a moderately severe dose. It is often the stage between acute and chronic.
- Chronic: refers to lingering, lasting exposure or to frequently occurring small dosages.

- Sensitization: People may become sensitive to a variety of substances. The sensitization process makes a person react to the toxic or chemical effects of a substance at much lower concentrations than before it occurred.

The chronic effects of exposure can be brought about in two main ways. An acute dosage can produce physiological effects that can linger on for long periods; small, repeated doses can produce similar effects over a period of time.

The wide range of effects noted in crib deaths requires a poison that can produce a variety of such effects, over a variety of exposure periods, with varying concentrations. Ammonia is one such poison. It can be mildly irritating or fatal depending on both the dosage and the person being poisoned.

One dosage factor that could cause the difference noted in sex ratios of male to female crib death rates is their anatomically different voiding mechanisms. The trajectory of urine issuing from the erect penis of a tiny boy is quite different from that issuing from his differently endowed sister.

Size is another feature that causes differences in dosage. The effects of a chemical vary according to the weight of the victim. The smaller the victim, the smaller the dosage required to poison it. Now in crib death victims, there is a marked difference between the lighter babies and the heavier babies. A lighter baby of say less than 2500g (6 lbs.) is at least 40 percent lighter than one weighing 4000g (8.6 lbs.) or more. And the mortality rate for such small infants is many times that of the larger.

In the ammonia poisoning factor theory, the poison originates from broken-down urea. The closer the nostrils of the victim are to the source of the gas, the greater the dosage received. It is also a fact that the same low-weight babies are also shorter — and hence, are closer to the ammonia source than longer, heavier babies. More short babies die from crib death than long babies.

As development occurs, the exposure to ammonia decreases and the dose/lb. body weight exposure to ammonia decreases. It is hardly a surprising coincidence to find that crib deaths have decreased markedly by about 6 months of age.

Table 5. Body Length and Weight Percentage of Male Infants at Birth and Six Months

At birth	At six months
3% are less than 47cm (18.50 inches), weigh less than 2.3kg (5 lbs.)	are less than 64 cm (25.19 inches), weight 6.6kg (14.5 lbs.)
50% are about 51cm (20 inches), weigh about 3.5kg (7.7 lbs.)	are about 68cm (26.7 inches), weigh 8kg (17.6 lbs.)
3% are more than 55cm (21.6 inches), weigh more than 4.4kg (9.7 lbs.)	are more than 73 cm (28.7 inches), weigh 10kg (22 lbs.)

Sensitization

Sensitization to ammonia is a possibility. It is only mentioned here because, if it were correct, then the wide range of poisoning effects from ammonia would be considerably increased and this would make ammonia a much more dangerous chemical than it already appears.

The Baby's Sleep Pattern

Babies that are awake cannot endure the pungent smell of ammonia and soon let their parents know of their discomfort. Sleeping babies are unconscious to the odor from ammonia and, if anything, have their sleep state deepened by inhaling the gas. Should a baby be affected by an acute, but nonlethal, dose of ammonia, the alkaline corrosion of the upper respiratory passages, the stomach, and the lungs would alter the behavior pattern of the baby. This happens because the baby is in pain and finds it difficult to breathe and settle down to sleep.

The length of uninterrupted sleep is highly important as a factor in ammonia poisoning. The most dangerous condition for the infant is a long winter's night because everyone tends to sleep longer through long winter nights. The baby is not going to be awakened as long as it is asleep if only because it is too cold and too inconvenient to check a sleeping baby on a cold winter night. For maximum ammonia production from urea, bacteria from feces is required. Feces are not essential to the breakdown of urea, though the longer the period the infant is undisturbed, the more ammonia can be released. (I have not come across any figures relating to the presence of feces with crib death victims.)

The Mother

Typically the crib death mother is one that has been under considerable stress due to a variety of causes — including her economic status, youth, lack of education, and overcrowded living conditions. The fact that she succeeds so often should not be credited to the modern society that focuses its total lack of care upon its most important function, but to her dedication to motherhood under very difficult conditions. It is not surprising that typically her house is squalid or unsanitary, or that she goes to bed so tired that the infant she has mothered so well gets left unattended while she sleeps. When her problems increase due to the arrival of a second infant, is it any wonder that the crib death rate for these infants is higher than for the first-born? The mother, who will not attend free health clinics because of their patronizing attitude, is hardly likely to be visiting the doctor with her infant when she is required to pay full rates. Whatever the cause, it would seem that a society that can afford palaces of patching can ill afford to see the source of its life so poorly catered to.

Acute Poisoning

Acute ammonia poisoning leaves a number of tell-tale effects on the victim depending on the severity of the inhalation. If it were sufficient, it would cause death either through pulmonary edema (liquid in the lungs) or by causing respiration to stop through reflex action. In addition, the alkaline effects of inhaling the ammonia would be evident on the upper respiratory tract. There would be corrosion of the larynx and trachea and hemorrhages throughout the breathing system. Soaps would be made from the natural body fats. The fluid that would be caused to flow from the action of the ammonia on the mucus membranes would combine with the soap. Suds would be made by the air blowing through the mixture of fluid and soap so froth would be produced. The froth would often be blood tinged from hemorrhaging. I have not seen reference to froth issuing from the nostrils or mouth of near-miss victims. Therefore, it would seem that such froth formation comes about late in the exposure to ammonia. This is consistent with the amount of ammonia needed to saponify tissue. It is also consistent with a fatal, acute ammonia dose.

The alkaline fluid formed with the acute exposure would be swallowed. Such liquid has a sufficiently high pH to curdle milk. (A 1% solution has a pH in excess of 11.) Milk changes to insoluble curds at around a pH of 5 (47). In addition, the ammonia fluid would cause stenosis (a narrowing) of the stomach, the duodenum, and the jejunum. The esophagus and stomach would be inflamed. Vomiting would often occur as a result of the curdling and the narrowing of the stomach.

Subacute and Nonlethal Acute Poisoning

The range of effects of ammonia poisoning on the body's total functioning is so widespread that it is difficult to list the effects in detail. Those effects would cover breathing difficulties, pain and suffering difficulties, respiratory problems, and intestinal problems. Apart from the immediate effect of the ammonia on the body systems, the after-exposure effects would tend to be painful, dangerous, and of long duration. The behavior, growth, and development of the infant could also be affected by the long-lasting ill effects of ammonia exposure.

The immediate effects would be similar to those listed for the severe acute attack, except not so pronounced. The baby would be in pain. It would be restless and it would have a cough and sniffles. Frequent vomiting and diarrhea could be expected. Difficulty in breathing because of constriction of the pharynx and lesions to the vocal cord would be expected. The cry of the baby would be altered due to damage to its vocal cords. The infant would tend to be cyanotic (bluish) because it would have difficulty breathing. Underventilation would be common and of long duration because of the damage to the lung tissue and because of the edema caused by ammonia inhalation. Such an exposure to a nonlethal acute or subacute dose could eventually prove fatal through the development of chemical pneumonitis. If pathogenic organisms were present in the damaged lung tissue, then it could be expected that a virulent infection would develop.

Severe apneic spells could be predicted because of spasm of the glottis or larynx caused by exposure to ammonia fumes.

Ammonia exposure causes temperature control problems. Thus, fever could be expected.

The damage caused to the alimentary canal would cause digestive and feeding problems. The infant would be irritable and would have difficulty digesting food. The fluid balance of the body would be upset. Thus, the infant would not thrive. It is important to note that both respiratory and gastroenteritis infant victims exhibit a periodicity of occurrence not unlike that of crib death victims. Diarrhea in infants is an extremely serious condition that could be caused by the curdling of the infant milk and by the effect of the ammonia on the infant gut. One of the features of diarrhea is that it is usually accompanied by vomiting. Infantile gastroenteritis usually occurs between the ages of 2 and 4 months. The condition is rare after 15 months of age. The precise cause is not known, although *E. coli* bacteria strains are found in some cases. It is almost always confined to artificially fed babies and it is rare in breast-fed babies. Those infants who are breast-fed and do have diarrhea usually have less severe attacks (48). Tetany may appear in diarrhea victims as occasional spells of continuous muscular contractions of all muscles, (particularly the extensor muscles that extend or straighten out the parts (3) (44)). The clustering of infant gastroenteritis caused deaths is also very similar to the clustering found in crib death victims. The inability to find a satisfactory causative agent for most of the victims is also very similar to the crib death story.

Chapter Eleven

Respiration and Ammonia

The Chemical Effects of Ammonia Inhalation and Temperature on Respiration

The chemical inhalation effects of ammonia are underventilation, hypoxemia, and respiratory arrest. The effects of deficit degrees of temperature on respiration are at the lungs, body cells, and respiratory control center. (Deficit degrees measure the temperature difference between the infant's body and the environment.)

The oxygen control defects found in crib death victims predispose the victim to ammonia inhalation and temperature problems.

The crib death factors relating to respiratory factors are:

- Growth
- Vulnerable underdevelopment
- Compensatory tissue development

Ammonia inhalation affects each step of respiration. It causes problems at the:

- Lung gas exchange sites
- Body cell gas exchange site
- Arterial blood oxygenation level
- Central control sites in the brain stem

Chronic, or long-term, underventilation and chronic hypoxemic symptoms are the two most common crib death autopsy features that defy explanation. (Hypoxemia is an oxygen deficiency in the bloodstream.) They point to respiratory failure as the basic cause of crib death. They also point to a long-term problem causing the respiratory failure. Steinschneider's apnea theory seems to be the answer here. A great deal of research has gone into his theory, but it still fails to account for the four-fifths of crib death victims who showed no previous history of apnea. The mechanical blocking of air from getting to the lung and into the bloodstream has long been offered as a cause of crib death. And indeed, features such as soft pillows and fluffy mattresses have been shown to cause asphyxiation. The *Medical Journal of Australia* recently published a letter that showed a fluffy sheepskin link to a crib death case in Tasmania. Internal blocking by the pharynx has been shown to be a cause of underventilation. Again these theories fail to account for the more than 50 percent of crib death victims who show chronic signs of underventilation and hypoxemia.

The poisoning effects of ammonia have been described. A number of these have relevance to respiration. Acute inhalation of ammonia causes respiratory arrest. It does this through causing pulmonary edema and through the damage it does to the lung capillary and lung alveolus membrane. Vomit, produced through the action of ammonia on the stomach and its contents, is sometimes sucked down the trachea into the lungs, causing pneumonia. The caustic damage to the upper respiratory tract causes a variety of responses that lead to underventilation. It causes spasms of the larynx or glottis. It is also able to produce a tightening, closing effect (stenosis) of the trachea. Its caustic action on the glottis and pharynx can cause edema and damage that will hinder breathing.

Quite aside from this variety of pathways through which ammonia directly or indirectly prevents oxygen intake by the bloodstream is the direct effect ammonia has on respiration itself.

It is through the direct chemical combination with carbon dioxide in the lungs and bloodstream that ammonia stops oxygen from being taken up or released by the blood and so directly causes hypoxemia and eventually respiratory arrest. To clarify this, it is necessary to go into some detail on the exchange of gases, their control, and the effect of carbon dioxide imbalance on respiration.

The exchange of respiratory gases takes place because of pressure differences between the gases in the air (lung alveoli) and the blood (lung capillaries). The term "partial pressure" and its symbol "P" are used to describe the concentration of a gas in a mixture of gases. Because the air in the lung spaces is only completely renewed every four or five breaths, the lung alveolar air is a different mixture from the outside air. It has a very much higher carbon dioxide concentration and a considerably lower oxygen concentration. It is also saturated with water vapor. The partial pressures for each of the gases in mm Hg, in dry air, alveolar air, and lung capillary blood are noted in the table that follows.

Table 6. Partial Pressures for Each of the Gases Contained in Dry Air, Alveolar Air and Lung Capillary Blood (49)

Gas	Pressure		
	Dry Air (mm Hg)	Alveolar Air (mm Hg)	Lung Capillary Blood (mm Hg)
P N$_2$	600	573	57
P O$_2$	15q (21%)	100 (14%)	40
P CO$_2$	0.3 (0.04%)	4.0 (5.5%)	45
P H$_2$O	0	47	47

It is important to note that a good deal of energy is required to heat and saturate with moisture cold dry air before it reaches the alveoli. A problem facing the infant when it is put down to sleep in a cold, dry room could be the deficit degree shock it receives. It could be enough to cause the infant to gasp and perhaps induce an apneic spell. In addition, the infant breathes at a shallow and rapid rate of from 30 to 40 breaths per minute, compared with the adult breathing rate of between 12 and 18 breaths per minute. Any temperature drop could depress the normal volume of inspired air per minute, and that would lower the oxygen available for respiration.

Blood gases in the lung capillaries have to be exchanged with air-gas mixtures in the alveoli. In order to coordinate blood rates, inhalation and exhalation rates, and alveolar air exchange rates, there has to be local control. There are such controls. If there are not enough local areas of oxygenated alveoli, the oxygen lack causes vasoconstriction to stop blood flowing into those areas where it wouldn't be able to exchange oxygen. If there are local areas where blood isn't flowing and there is a low level of carbon dioxide, broncho-constriction will occur to reduce the flow of air into such a space. It is not difficult to foresee the havoc that could be created in such a finely tuned local system, if a gas that combined directly with the carbon dioxide of the air were introduced. It is precisely that chemical reaction that ammonia causes because it combines directly with carbon dioxide in the presence of water vapor.

There is an additional respiratory center effect of such a drop in carbon dioxide level in the lungs. A well-known trick used by underwater swimmers is to hyperventilate before diving into the water. The deep breathing removes carbon dioxide from the lung air, and the need-to-breathe reflex is stopped. Therefore, the underwater swimmer can swim a lot farther without feeling the need to breathe. The only problem is that this sometimes proves to be fatal because the swimmer may drown by becoming unconscious.

The point to be stressed is that the breathing switch is not activated by a lack of oxygen, but by the level of free carbon dioxide present.

The cessation of the breathing reflex, caused for the diver by his diluting his lung carbon dioxide, is an artificially caused apneic spell brought about by the drop in the concentration of the carbon dioxide.

The gases present in the bloodstream are not carried as simple solutions of the gas in the blood. There is very little oxygen carried in solution. Nearly all of it is carried in chemical combination with the blood as oxyhemoglobin. There are three factors which allow or hinder the release of the oxygen from the oxyhemoglobin. Two of these controls have particular relevance to the crib death theory. They are the temperature effect and the carbon dioxide concentration effect. The third factor is the partial pressure of the oxygen.

Oxygen is released from the oxyhemoglobin if there is a high concentration of carbon dioxide in the arterial blood (for example, after strenuous exercise). If the carbon dioxide level is lowered, then the oxygen is held by the oxyhemoglobin and not released to the tissues. Because ammonia is able to reduce the carbon dioxide level of the lungs and blood, it reduces the concentration of the carbon dioxide, and so the body is starved of oxygen. The result can be chronic underventilation, hypoxemia, and respiratory arrest.

The other factor controlling the release of oxygen from the oxyhemoglobin is the temperature. Any body temperature buildup through exercise allows extra oxygen to be made available to the cells of the body for respiration. Having such a temperature-sensitive system for rationing out the needed oxygen molecules, as and where needed, is a very neat system indeed as it does not need central control. A body temperature drop also has a dramatic effect on the release of oxygen from the oxyhemoglobin. It is this effect that is widely used in the treatment of head surgery and in cardiac surgery to artificially cause a drop in the body temperature and thus reduce the oxygen consumption by the tissues.

Crib deaths are much more frequent in cold, wintry conditions than in hot, humid countries and seasons. Since hypothermia symptoms have been shown to be agents of underventilation and as a number of infants have exhibited temperature-control irregularities prior to death, respiratory arrest through long periods of deficit degrees could be a significant cause of respiratory arrest and death.

The effect of chronic deficit degrees of temperature is the condition called hypothermia. Now hypothermia victims exhibit a wide range of behavioral differences from people with normal temperature. So the deficit degree factor has an influence and effect in the brain as well as throughout the body. Such a central respiratory effect of deficit degrees on infant monkeys has been shown. Infant monkeys with cold or wet stimuli to the cheek became apneic and developed a slow rate of heartbeat within seconds.

A decrease in the arterial carbon dioxide partial pressure (concentration) leads to chronic or long-term, effects on the brain. Ventilation is so exquisitely sensitive to changes in $P\ CO_2$, that a small decrease in $P\ CO_2$ offsets much of the ventilatory stimulation that hypoxia might otherwise cause. It takes a day or so to recover from a decrease in $P\ CO_2$. (50) Since the respiratory drive is produced by the action of carbon dioxide inside the center — and not the oxygen level — the decrease in drive produced by the low $P\ CO_2$ will lead to a decrease in the ventilatory response to the oxygen lack itself and so will cause underventilation, hypoxemia, and respiratory arrest. In addition, the ventilatory response is reduced by various drugs that depress the respiratory center — for example, morphine and barbiturates. The ventilatory response is also reduced if there are any factors causing the work of breathing to be increased.

Respiration — The Oxygen Problem

There is considerable evidence that a large number of infants are born with oxygen deficiency problems. The underdeveloped, light-weight baby often results from an inadequate oxygen supply during pregnancy.

It has already been noted that the oxygen dissociated from oxyhemoglobin is affected by temperature, oxygen supply, and carbon dioxide. Fetal blood has a similar oxyhemoglobin dissociation system, but the oxygen is bound more firmly than in adult oxyhemoglobin. With the fetal blood having greater affinity for oxygen, the oxygen will tend to leave the maternal and enter the fetal blood, and so at a given oxygen pressure, the fetal blood becomes more saturated than the maternal blood. (46) The firmer binding of the oxygen in the fetus presents no problem for the fetus, provided the blood supply of the mother is adequate. Problems arise when the mother is anemic or a smoker. Then the mother's blood is inadequately oxygenated and so the fetal blood is inadequately oxygenated. Thus, the whole fetal development is limited and the infant is born at term underweight, underventilated, and chronically hypoxemic. After birth, the fetal type of hemoglobin gradually disappears and is replaced by the adult type. Therefore, some children start life having for months suffered from an oxygen deficiency. This deficiency has not only resulted in stunted overall body development, as the fetal brain stem has a higher metabolic rate than other areas of the brain, the brain stem with its respiratory control center is particularly affected by a chronic lack of oxygen. There is a continuation of fetal blood production centers found in more than half of the crib death victims. It appears that the fetal blood persists in these infants. So such infants would suffer more from lack of oxygen than infants who had passed from the phase of fetal blood production to postnatal blood production.

It has already been noted that the respiratory process in lung gas transfer, in arterial and body cell transport and transfer, and in central respiratory control are all tuned into a system controlled by the carbon dioxide concentration. This is not a total control system as there are oxygen chemoreceptor systems throughout the respiratory system and in particular in the carotid tissues that have a feedback oxygen respiration control function. However, the level of gas control and respiratory control is on a gross oxygen deficit scale, compared to the fine tuning of the carbon dioxide and temperature control. Furthermore, the analysis of crib death victim symptoms points to a deficiency in development of the carotid bodies in more than half the dead infants. Thus, their oxygen respiratory control is even more limited than it normally would be.

Crib death infant autopsy surveys have discovered a large number of chronic responses by the infant to survive in a poisoned atmosphere. One must remember not to view the crib death victim as a 3-week-old baby or a 4-month-old baby, but as a 10-month-old to 14-month-old person. And viewed from that perspective, even the lack of size of many infants is a response to the lack of oxygen they experienced in their uterine development. Perhaps if the woman who smoked was made to realize that she was slowly poisoning her yet-to-be born infant in a womb that doesn't nourish, then she might stop smoking so excessively. Perhaps if she realized more clearly that her fetal prisoner, entombed in her womb, nourished only through her placenta, can emerge crippled through oxygen starvation and inadequate dietary nourishment, she would be a better mother.

Viewed from this perspective, the infant's excessive tissue development of pulmonary arterial muscle, cardiac right ventricles, brown fat, adrenal gland, cortisone, brain stem, scavenger cells, and more are the desperate organic adaptations of the infant to cope with a hostile environment—an environment lacking one of its most essential elements: oxygen.

Chapter Twelve

A Lethal Hypothesis

Many sudden infant deaths have been shown to be not unexpected. But the deaths are almost invariably silent. How did my limp son sleep through the pungent concentration of ammonia that jerked my head back? Limpness is a feature almost invariably noted with these deaths, as is also the evidence of a relaxed bladder. Then there are the animal experiments with ammonia. Rats have been exposed. They went into a coma and died. Lesser concentrations sent them into a coma from which they appeared to recover as though nothing had happened after exposure ceased.

The hypothesis is that ammonia may act on sleeping infants as a lethal anesthetising agent. Many low-weight gases and volatile liquids are very potent anesthetising agents. Ammonia is a lethal gas. There is considerable evidence that can be drawn from the environmental conditions, the pre-death infant symptoms, and the postmortem clinical state of sudden death infants to support this hypothesis. In low concentrations, the effect on the whole infant body would be the most important consideration until anoxia became critical. For then the anesthetic effect of the ammonia would become the deciding factor.

The ability of ammonia to cause a localized respiratory obstruction, laryngitis, or epiglottitis is compelling. But against acute laryngeal obstruction — as every clinician knows — is the noise of laryngitis and the general consensus is that S.I.D.S. is silent.

So there is silent death. There is no laryngeal stridor. There is limpness. How can these facts be related to ammonia exposure? At a local level, ammonia has effects on the skin. It can cause severe diaper rash, and internally it inflames the mucus membranes of the respiratory and the digestive tracts. In a general way, it can affect the whole body. It can cause chronic underventilation, hypoxemia, and respiratory arrest by its direct effect on carbon dioxide, the respiratory control mechanism.

Apart from causing these effects by removing carbon dioxide from the respiratory tract, the respiratory drive produced by the central nervous system is chronically affected. The decrease in drive produced by the low P CO_2 will lead to a decrease in the ventilatory response to the oxygen lack itself and will reinforce the underventilation, the hypoxemia, and the respiratory arrest.

The essential, or central, site of action then is the central nervous system, where a chemical anesthetising agent and hypoxemia are acting in tandem. This chemical anesthetic, rather than the mechanical laryngeal spasm or edema obstruction, is the real danger. A degree of respiratory obstruction or respiratory difficulty or inadequacy is produced.

The breathing response of rib cage and diaphragm becomes ineffective due to the general limpness also induced (hypotonia of muscles). Perhaps during a Rapid Eye Movement sleep stage, the general anoxia may cross the transition point where increasing anoxia leads to less, rather than more, respiratory effort. The question of Rapid Eye Movement sleep is interesting, in that if one is deprived of it, it becomes compulsive so the infant could be driven to the point of no return. Thus, an essentially toxic, poisonous anesthetic death takes place.

The descriptions of autopsy findings and the postmortem clinical state of the sudden death infants are consistent with such an anesthetic death.

Chapter Thirteen

The Nonspecific Environmental Stress Trauma Exposure Profile

While trying to warn mothers of the dangers facing their infants, I am filled with bleak, crushing depression as I contemplate the lot of so many infants born into our so-called advanced society. I grieve for the needless loss of infants who are dying because of the evil influence modern society has on them — the influence of an advertising system that seduces young people to poison themselves and their offspring with smoking, alcohol, and drugs — an advertising system that can continue to operate without having to pay a cent for the devastation it causes — a system that even gets subsidized by the state to continue with its advertising so the death-causing sales may increase.

I grieve for the infants born to die because society makes the young mother and her family the economic outcasts and the losers in a race for material goods. She and her family are left unsupported and uncared for, as the lowest order of society, fit only for its crumbs.

I grieve for the infants who are born to die because their mothers have been conditioned all their lives to regard their breasts solely as sexual adornments — never to be disfigured by the trauma of nursing an infant for more than a token time.

I grieve for the infant who has been starved of oxygen in the uterus and who when born is refused the only food specifically designed to combat infection and promote optimum health and growth. Instead, this baby is force-fed the poison of so-called infant formula foods and dies of "unknown causes" from gastroenteritis.

I grieve for the helpless infant born into a society that glories in its annual multibillion dollar "health" budget. This budget is designed to cure the ill effects of the success of the advertising of products that are poisoning the society. We live in a society that pays a token amount to prevent easily avoided destruction — a society with huge vested interests in not preventing death.

It is important to try to cover all possibilities when discussing the effects of a poison. However, it's extremely difficult to fully establish just how far ammonia's ill effects extend, for ammonia has quite an incredible range of ill effects. And the ill effects themselves are so variable from person to person.

I became interested in the chronic effects of ammonia when I realized they could cause both pneumonia and diarrhea with vomiting. I became even more interested when I found that both diseases, and related ones, exhibit a periodicity quite similar to that of crib death. Then I read that, in a number of places throughout the Western world, there has been a decline in the number of recorded crib death cases over a period of years. Then I read how Urquhart and his co-workers published their observations that the antiglobulin antibody had been found in half the 39 instances of sudden infant death and half of the eight deaths due to respiratory or gastrointestinal infection. On the other hand, the antibody was found in only 5 percent of the 21 living controls with a variety of inflammatory processes.

It was apparent that a pattern was again emerging — a pattern that rationalized the role of ammonia poisoning into acute and chronic classes. It could be possible that crib death victims were mainly acute cases of ammonia exposure and respiratory deaths were chronic effects.

Then I examined a variety of graphs showing crib deaths and pneumonia deaths plotted against the months in which they occurred (12, 53). Also I found an age distribution graph for crib deaths and for all respiratory deaths in England and Wales. This graph shows extremely similar curves with no statistically significant differences between the two distributions; nor was there any difference in the age distribution of boys and girls (13). Put another way, there was a total statistical relationship between the crib death and pulmonary death infants, in both age and sex distribution numbers.

The graph on the next page is from data supplied by the New Zealand National Health Statistics Center in Wellington.

The graph data is for post-neonatal deaths (one month through one year) in New Zealand in 1978 through '79. The graph confirms the statistical relationship between crib death and respiratory and intestinal causes. Nervous disorders, circulatory disease, metabolic and immunity disorders, as well as neoplastic, endocrinal, nutritional, infectious, and parasitic dis-

Death Cause Relationships in Post-neonatal Infants

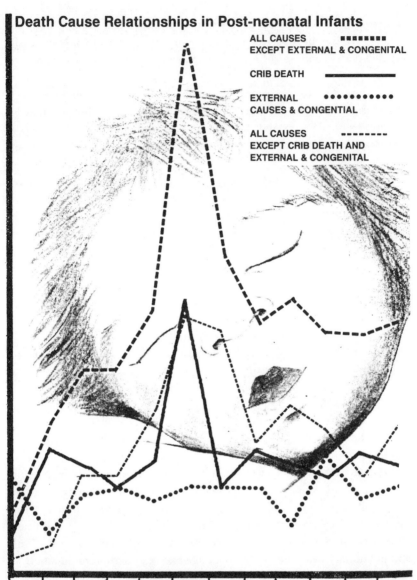

ALL CAUSES ■■■■■■■■
EXCEPT EXTERNAL & CONGENITAL

CRIB DEATH ▬▬▬▬▬

EXTERNAL ●●●●●●●●●●●
CAUSES & CONGENTIAL

ALL CAUSES ▬ ▬ ▬ ▬ ▬
EXCEPT CRIB DEATH AND
EXTERNAL & CONGENITAL

JAN FEB MAR APRIL MAY JUNE JULY AUG SEPT OCT NOV DEC

**Post-neonatal infant (1m – 1yr) deaths
In N.Z. 1978 – 1979 by month of death.**

THE N.E.S.T.* EXPOSURE PROFILE
ACUTE AND CHRONIC LETHAL EXPOSURE GRAPH
*Nonspecific Environmental Stress Trauma

orders were included because all the symptoms are compatible in one way or another with the chronic effect symptoms of ammonia poisoning. The only two major categories that could definitely be excluded from any ammonia consideration would be deaths from accidents or external cause and congenital deaths.

The relationship between sudden crib death victims and the total of the remainder is clear if crib death is viewed as primarily exhibiting acute symptoms and the remainder as exhibiting chronic symptoms of exposure to nonspecific environmental stress trauma.

A detailed description of gastroenteritis symptoms and their relationship to crib death symptoms has already been given. However, it is interesting to note the similarity of symptoms between pneumonia or respiration disease and chronic ammonia poisoning.

Anatomic differentiation of pneumonia is of no value in childhood. Causative organisms are often difficult to isolate in small children (39). In many instances, the usual pathogenic organisms have not been isolated from the sick child. Also the course of the disease is not altered by sulphonamide or antibacterial therapy. There is a great variation of symptoms, depending upon the age of the child. Vomiting, diarrhea, prostration and toxemia, cough, dyspnea, cyanosis, restlessness, muscular pains, headache, chest pain, chills, respiratory distress with increased shallow respirations and movements of the alae nasae, expiratory grunt, convulsions and other signs of meningeal irritation may be present in variable amounts. The onset may be abrupt or it may follow symptoms of an upper respiratory infection. Acute bronchiolitis and interstitial pneumonitis are used interchangeably especially in pulmonary infections of infants (48). Such a vast array of symptoms certainly could be masking an ammonia factor involvement.

Although ammonia poisoning and its multitude of phantom effects could be a primary cause, there is too distinct and clear a relationship between gastroenteritis and artificial feeding, as well as other factors for it to be the sole cause.

Studies, demonstrating that apneic response to chemical laryngeal stimulation—with cow milk, for example—is enhanced when test animals' central respiratory drive is depressed, are possible pointers to a combination of factors involving artificial food. There are far too many symptoms found in the infant of anaphylactic shock to be confident of a simple answer. But, at very least, the ammonia factor theory provides a positive framework wherein the limits of each causative factor can be traced given sufficient data. The predictive nature of the ammonia factor system is one of the clearest indicators of its validity.

A final sobering thought is that if ammonia poisoning, in all its varied disguises, causes deaths in so many neonatal babies, what long-term effects must be caused in those who do not die from such exposure, but survive?

Chapter Fourteen

N.E.S.T. Exposure Prevention

Because the large number of possible environmental stress traumas that can afflict infants have similar (nonthriving) nonspecific effects on those infants, it is extremely difficult to quantify a particular stress trauma effect. The N.E.S.T. exposure graph gives a clue to the possible solution to this problem. The graph can represent a chronic and an acute picture of stress that in turn represents a deficiency problem. This problem has to do with the absence of essential parts of the infant's life requirements. The main inputs for the infant are food and respiratory gases. Under a regimen of mainly artificial feeding and non-breast milk, it is easy to envision a situation where essential human infant requirements are not supplied despite what so-called research and milk companies would like us to believe. Ammonia production has been quite clearly linked to the artificial food regime. The fact that non-Caucasian races have a much higher infant death rate than Caucasians would seem to indicate a possible artifical, European, cow-milk digestion problem. It could indicate a large number of other specific sensitivities too.

Ammonia, of course, could interfere with the availability of carbon dioxide. This gas is so exquisitely in control of the respiration process that any alteration in its availability for the infant poses major problems. I have a detailed description from a New Zealand mother that may provide some interesting lines of procedure. Her infant seemed at one stage to produce exceptionally smelly urine. She found the baby one night apparently lifeless. Through heart massage and mouth-to-mouth resuscitation, the infant revived. It's possible that, if the infant's breathing had been cut off by the removal of carbon dioxide, the input of carbon dioxide through the mother's efforts might have been the breathing restart switch. This would seem to indicate that a small percentage of carbon dioxide should be included in those respiratory gases given to infants who are struggling to breathe. Once the carbon dioxide control has turned off the breathing process, no amount of straight oxygen or possibly straight compressed air can revive the infant. The example also demonstrates how important it is for every mother or parent to be given actual training in resuscitation.

Little specific research has taken place in terms of collecting detailed possible environmental trauma evidence. This has resulted in a major problem in determining N.E.S.T. exposure. There seems to be some glaring gaps. Medicines, drugs, and chemical exposure require much more investigation. The available data is deficient not only for sudden infant death cases, but especially for the respiratory disease and gastrointestinal disease death groups.

Because any possible death factor that was evenly spread across the infant death profile was systematically excluded from the lavishly funded crib death research projects, a new overview of all accompanying causative death factors is necessary.

Any model for the prevention of infant death needs to take into account the totality of the sociological and environmental factors associated with the death, as well as the development of the infant. Because infant deaths are not found with any specific medical conditions and are found with a wide variety of symptoms, particular attention must be placed on avoiding environmental stress trauma exposure.

Selye showed that *combinations* of environmental stresses can be lethal, even though single stresses are not. In experiments with rats subjected to chemical irritation on their skin and immobilized by being bound up, there was a dramatically increased mortality rate over those rats subjected to chemical skin irritation only (54).

It must be remembered that, when an infant is born, it is subjected to a wide variety of stressful environmental changes. Indeed, some birth experiences are so traumatic that the infant suffers stress for long periods after birth. The new process of breathing air, temperature variation exposure, wearing clothes, being handled, movement restriction, oral feeding, digestion, defecation, rashes, germs, and viruses are all possible sources of stress.

In addition, maternal stress has been shown to be an environmental factor that increases the liability of the infant to crib death.

It could be questioned whether high-cost apnea alarms are helpful in preventing crib deaths. It has not been shown that arrested periods of breathing are a cause of crib death. The high-cost monitors hardly justify their extensive use. A possible alternative is a wet diaper warning mechanical device. It would also have the advantage of being quite cheap. With this device, there is positive assurance that all is well with the infant. It also ensures that the infant is comfortable. In addition, this device could warn of any near-miss situation. It is a fact that crib death infants have wet diapers, although it has not been established whether the infant wets its diaper after death or preceding it.

The nonspecific environmental stress trauma exposure model of infant death provides predictive, protective, causative, and preventative elements to a model that originated in the realization that a deadly poisonous gas was potentially present at every crib. Ammonia is a lethal environmental hazard that had not previously been checked by the medical profession. It provides a model that does not require implementation by the medical profession. It provides a model calling for the improved environment of infants. It will base its research on the cooperation of parents. It is a model that focuses on the hazardous impact of adverse environmental conditions on the infant. It is a model of educational welfare and infant care. Acceptance of the theory would lead in time to a vigorous program of preventive re-education for parents in order to prevent these deaths and have healthier infants.

References

1. Tyler J., *Cot Death: The Ammonia Factor*, J. Tyler, Hokianga, New Zealand, 1983

2. Carpenter R.G., Gardner A., Pursall E., McWeeny P.M., Emery J.L., Identification of some infants at immediate risk of dying unexpectedly and justifying intensive care. Lancet, August 18, 1979

3. Thomson W.A., Editor. Black's Medical Dictionary 32nd edition, 1979

4. Naeye R.L., "Sudden infant death." Scientific American.
   Vol 240 pgs 52-58 1980.

5. Beckwith J.B., "The sudden infant death syndrome." Curr Probl Pediat. 3(8) : 1973.

6. Spiers P.S., "Estimated rates of concordancy for the sudden infant death syndrome in twins." American Epidemiological Journal 100 (1) : 1974.

7. Valdes-Dapena, Marie., "Sudden Unexplained infant death 1970-1975. An evolution in understanding."
   Pathology Annual Vol 12 p11 pps 114-165, 1977.

8. Fohlin, Proceedings of the Francis E. Camps international symposium on sudden and unexpected death in Infancy. Toronto, Ontario, Canada 1974.

9. Steele R., "Sudden infant death syndrome in Ontario, Canada. Epidemiological aspects." From *Proceedings of the second international conference on causes of sudden death in infants*.

10. Fraser J. (editor), "Post Neonatal infant mortality survey. Results of a National survey 1978-79." National Health Statistics Centre 1981.

11. Kraus J.F., Borhani N.O., "Post neonatal, sudden unexpected death in California. A cohort study."
    American Epidemiological Journal
    95: 497 1972.

12. Tonkin S.L., "Epidemiology of SIDS in Auckland, New Zealand" in Robinson R.R. (editor)
    S.I.D.S. 1974 Toronto
    Canadian Foundation for the study of infant deaths. 1974.

13. Camps F.E., Carpenter R.G. (Editors)
    Sudden and unexpected deaths in infancy (cot-deaths)
    Bristol, Wright 1972.

14. Holy. Pg 101 Session 4 of Sudden and unexpected deaths in infancy (cot-deaths) edited by Camps F.E. and Carpenter R.G.

15. Bergman A.B., Ray C.G., Pomeroy M.A., Wahl P.W., Beckwith J.B. "Studies of the sudden infant death syndrome in King Country Washington"
    Pediatrics 49 (6) : 860 1972.
16. Froggatt P., Lynas M.A., Marshall T.K.,
    "Sudden unexpected death in infants (cot-deaths) Report of a collaborative study in Northern Ireland."
    Ulster Medical Journal 40:116 1971.
17. Stanton, A.N., "Overheating and cot-death" Lancet, November 24, 1984, pp 1199-1201
18. *The Health Consequences of smoking for women.* A report of the surgeon general. Washington D.C. Dept of Health and Human Services. 1980.
19. Pierson D.S., Howard P., Kleber H.,
    "Sudden deaths in infants born to methadone-maintained addicts."
    J.A.M.A. 220 (13) 1733 1972.
20. Child Health and Child Health Services in New Zealand. B. of Health Report Series No. 31
21. Sattaur O., Wet nappies could cause cot deaths. New Scientist 5 Jan 1984.
22. "New Zealand Mortality and Demographic Data Report," 1979, National Health Statistics Centre, Wellington, New Zealand.
23. Valman, Bernard., "Preventing Infant Deaths," *British Medical Journal* Volume 290. pp 339-340
24. Tonkin S.C., Stewart J.H., Withy S.,
    "Obstruction of the upper airway as a mechanism of sudden infant death. Evidence for a restricted nasal airway contributing to pharyngeal obstruction."
    Sleep. 3 (3/4) 375-382 Raven Press 1980.
25. Swift P.G.F. and Emery J.L., "Clinical observations on response to nasal occlusion in infancy." Arch. Dis Child 18 : 947-51 1973.
26. Carpenter, R.G., "Role of infection, suffocation and bottle feeding in cot-death." From Proceedings on the conference of sudden death in infancy. Sept. 1963, Seattle
27. Mars H., "Biogenic amine metabolism in apnea and crib death." from Hasselmeyer E.G., *Research prospectus in the sudden infant death syndrome.* D.H.E.W. Publication no NHI 76-1976.
28. Steinschneider A. Prolonged apnea and the sudden infant death syndrome. Clinical and laboratory observations.
    Pediatrics 50 : 646 1972.

29. Guntheroth W.G., "Fundamentals of clinical cardiology. Sudden infant death syndrome (crib death)" *American Heart Journal* June 1977, Vol 93 No 6.

30. Emery J.L. and Black M.M. "Apnea and Unexpected Child death." Report of the conference at Sheffield July 1979.
Lancet August 18, 1979.

31. Naeye R.L., Drage J. "Sudden infant death syndrome. A prospective study."
Ped. Res. g 298 Abstract 1975.

32. Patrick J.R., "Cardiac or Respiratory death?" Pg 130-132 in S.I.D.S. Proceedings of the 2nd International Conference on Causes of Sudden Death in Infants 1969 — edited by Bergman A.B. Beckwith J.B. and Ray C.G. University of Washington Press.

33. Beckwith J.B. as for (25). Pg 132.

34. Farber S., "Fulminating streptococcus infections in infancy as a cause of sudden death." New England Medical Journal
211 : 154 1934.

35. Naeye R.L., Drage J., "Sudden infant death syndrome. A prospective study." Ped Res 9 : 298. Abstract 1975 and So.Ped.Res.
Proceedings of the Meeting Amer.Ped.Soc. Denver April 16-19 1975.

36. Emery J.L., Gadson D.R., "Neural fat in the brains of infants dying in the perinatal period and presenting as unexpected death in infancy." Scientific program of the Pathological Society of Great Britain and Ireland Jan 9-11 1975 London.

37. Adelson L., "Specific studies of infant victims of sudden death." Proceedings in the conference on causes of sudden death in infants. Sept. 1963 Seattle.
Editors: R.J. Wedgwood and E.P. Benditt.

38. N. Roper Editor.
Nurses Dictionary 15th Edition.
Churchill, Livingstone 1978.

39. Marshall, P.D, "Pulmonary oedema"
British Journal of Diseases of the Chest. 1980 : Vol 74. pp 2-22

40. Gleason et al., *Clinical toxicology of commercial products*. Williams and Wilkins Co. 1969.

41. Braker W. and Siegel D.,
Effects of exposure to toxic gases. First aid and Medical treatment
2nd Edition 1977 Matheson.

42. Patty F.A. Editor,
    Vol II Toxicology of Industrial Hygiene and toxicology
    (in three vols)
    2nd revised edition 1963
    Interscience publishers.

43. Silver, Kempe, Briyn,
    Handbook of Pediatrics 10th Edition
    Lange 1973.

44. Gunther W., Discussion Pg 15
    Sudden and unexpected deaths in infancy (cot-deaths)
    Edited by Camps F.E. and Carpenter G 1972.

45. Seely S, "COUP de Grass?"
    Article in Guardian Newspaper, Manchester, England
    14.10.1982.

46. Tanner J.M., Whitehouse R.H.,
    "Height and weight charts from birth to five years, allowing for length
    of gestation." Arch Dis. Child 48, 786 1973.

47. Fruton & Simmonds,
    Pg 102 *General Biochemistry 2nd Edition*, John Wiley & Sons 1959.

48. Benz G.S., *Pediatric Nursing 4th Edition*
    C.V. Mosby Co St Louis 1960.

49. Chaffee and Lytle,
    Basic Physiology and Anatomy 4th Edition, Lippincourt 1980.

50. Mines A.H.,
    Respiratory physiology Raven Press Series in Physiology 1981.

51. Rafter, P. Never let go. Published 1972.

52. Taylor, S. Private communication 1984.

53. NHSC Job request P.N.S. 04 for TYLER, Post Neonatal Survey 1978-
    79 Race of Mother by cause of infant death, Sex, month of death.
    10.6.83.

54. Selye, Hans, *The Stress of Life* McGraw Hill Book Co. 1956

Index

1219

618.92 Tyler, James W.
TYI
　　　Sudden infant death
　　　(S. I. D. S.)

$ 5. 95　　　　　　　3

DATE			

1219